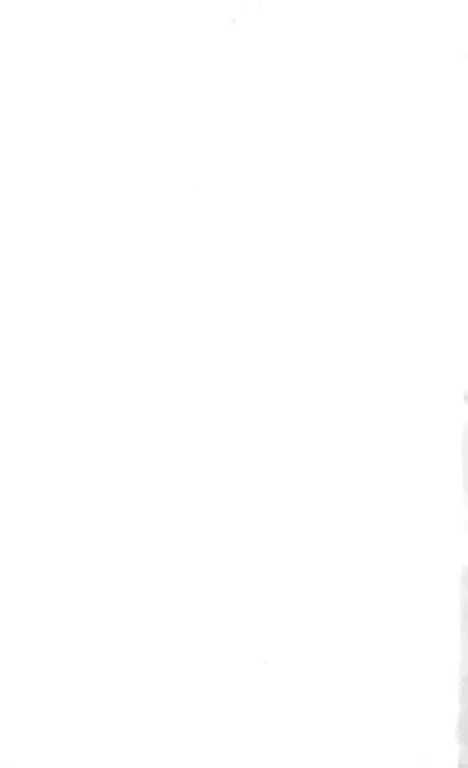

Pleneurethic: Way of Life, System of Therapeutics

PLENEURETHIC:
Way of Life,
System of Therapeutics

Richard Bangs Collier

Exposition Press   Hicksville, New York

ACKNOWLEDGMENTS

I wish to thank Iris Myers, Margaret Spackman, Robert W. Shields, Suni Telan, Joseph E. Hotung, and Nancy Frasco. Without their help this condensation of the original eight volumes of *Pleneurethic* would not have been possible. I am also grateful to Ravin V. Korothy, the editor of this book, for her expert professional assistance.   —R.B.C.

Pleneurethic is listed by Cornell and Indiana universities as a recent philosophical publication. It is also listed by *Philosophy,* journal of the Royal Institute of Philosophy (London, Cambridge University Press), and *Philosophy and Phenomenological Research,* journal of the International Phenomenological Society (Buffalo, State University of New York). *Science,* official journal of the American Association for the Advancement of Science, listed volume 6 of *Pleneurethic* in its May 26, 1972, edition.

FIRST EDITION

© 1979 by Richard Bangs Collier

Library of Congress Catalog Card Number: 79-50658

ISBN 0-682-49372-4

Printed in the United States of America

CONTENTS

PREFACE

This book hardly scratches the surface of the total field of Pleneurethic as outlined in the original eight-volume work *Pleneurethic* (Hong Kong, South China Morning Post Ltd., 1963-1972), of which it is a spartan condensation.

Numerous people have asked me to teach the art and practice of Pleneurethic. I have resolutely refused to do this, even though a large sum of money was offered me on one occasion.

Acceptance of the scientific and philosophical principles of Pleneurethic on academic levels must precede my teaching of its practice. Once the merit of Pleneurethic has been recognized by universities, then the way will be cleared for courses in the practice of its art.

The only alternative to this is the establishment of a state or federal law licensing the practice of Pleneurethic, and limiting such practice to doctors of Pleneurethic, graduated from colleges of Pleneurethic. These colleges would have clinics or hospitals where instruction in the practice of Pleneurethic would take place, and where students would train to pass state Pleneurethic examinations.

Pleneurethic: Way of Life, System of Therapeutics

INTRODUCTION

Pleneurethic is a way of life and system of therapeutics based on a balanced view of the whole person, and the several environments which encompass that person.

If we would understand Pleneurethic we must understand the capabilities and limitations of the central neural system, more specifically the brain. Pleneurethic integrates the vast field of human affairs by relating all things to brain capability.

On a biological level, Pleneurethic postulates the brain as the center of our being. The brain accumulates tension and reacts according to the aggregate. It must dissipate this tension or retain the accumulation and absorb the deleterious consequences.

Man's well-being is also dependent upon the soundness of his structure. Structural distortion produces functional abnormality that in turn is the cause of health problems, both mental and physical.

Pleneurethic seeks to preserve structural integrity to foster the biological basis for spontaneous health. If distortion occurs in one structural system, correlative distortions occur sympathetically in collateral systems. This is true of the human body and mind. It is also true of social and political institutions.

Operative Pleneurethic, then, is concerned with mind, mentality, the somatic body, and all processes of life. In Pleneurethic we are not just a chemical person, or a spiritual person, or a psychological entity; rather, we are a whole person.

Speculative Pleneurethic looks to the structure of civilization and aspects of the universe within which the total person must function.

PLENEURETHIC—
WHAT IT IS

PART 1

The term *Pleneurethic* is derived from three basic words: *plenary,* meaning completely competent and with total authority; *neural,* relating to the brain; and *ethos* or *ethic,* having to do with responsible behavior and constructive conduct.

Thus, Pleneurethic is the school of thought that teaches the way of life compatible with complete cerebellar competence guided by an ethical and wise mentality.

It is also a discipline and system of therapeutics predicated on the idea that chronic dissatisfactions are caused by patterns of disorder in the brain.

Pleneurethic represents an integrated way of life, centering around one single universal value. It is an international system of relevant thought and ethical behavior aimed at improving world civilization. It seeks to achieve this by assisting the individual to become a better person physically and mentally through enlightened brain management.

On a broad scale, Pleneurethic sees life systems, and the environment within which life must survive, as a series of interrelated structures and substructures with the brain as the central biological structure. There are five sides, or facets, to any device in the universe: structure, function, content, input, and output. And in any such device of man or nature, structural design controls the span of function.

The simplest inanimate engine is a loop knot in a piece of string. The structure of the knot functions to shorten the string, increase its mass at the juncture of the knot and provide feedback monitoring of tension with tightening, because the string is reflected upon itself. The content of the knot is string. There is an input into the knot and an energy output, as opposite ends of the knot are manipulated.

Living creatures are also engines. They are structured to produce a function and are constructed of materials that constitute their content. They receive an input, produce an output, and are provided with feedback circuitry for control through monitoring of activity.

In man, as in all engines, excessive structural alteration may swing the range of function into a distorted area. It may adversely modify content and may even impair the body's ability to receive a normal input or transmit a normal output.

In fact, chance for structural distortion of an interlocking nature is greater in man than in less complicated life forms. Man is of a structure, within a structure, within yet another structure.

Pleneurethically speaking, disease and disability are categorized in three divisions: chronic, acute, and congenital.

Pleneurethic therapy is directed primarily to the first.

Chronic illness is an unrelenting process caused by degenerative disturbances to the central neural system, more specifically the brain. Chronic illnesses do not cure themselves with passage of time because the power of brain to coordinate body activity and cooperate with the mind has been chronically diminished.

Acute illnesses are caused by vectors other than those responsible for chronic brain disturbance. Acute illness is generally healed with passage of time because the central neurological resources of brain remain unharmed and virtually undiminished throughout the acute emergency.

Congenital abnormality derives from permanent brain defects occurring during gestation.

Brain competence is the prime reality of Pleneurethic. Hence mechanisms by which neural energy is generated, conserved, and expended in health and disease processes are of the utmost importance.

All chronic disabilities of man are diagnosed in terms of brain involvement, and all avenues of therapy are directed at relieving the cause of whatever brain debility exists.

The brain and the remainder of the central and peripheral neural system are enclosed in a protective environment of ducts termed by Pleneurethic—the bioductory system.

This system of ducts is flexible within limits and provides foramina for access by blood and lymph vessels.

It conducts and protects the neural system as it journeys to all parts of the body. It contains and transmits the nerves in much the same manner as the circulatory system funnels the blood, the pulmonary system channels the respiratory gases, and the digestive system mixes and pushes the food along, supplying it with proper juices en route.

The bioductory system surrounds the nerves and forms both osseous and soft tissue ducts through which the nerve tracts transit. It directly supports, shields, and aids the neural system.

The bioductory system, one of the most important anatomical structures in the body, was, prior to Pleneurethic, one of the least understood.

In fact, its existence as a system was not even recognized.

Pleneurethic conceives the coaxiality of the bioductory system and the neural system as being of mechanical nature and vulnerable to physical abuse and trauma. The brain, too, is believed to be coaxial with the mentality of the mind. Triaxiality, in Pleneurethic, recognizes the complex situation of the brain being influenced chronically by mechanical bioductory derangement from injury and acutely by mental malstructure of the mind.

Bioductory trauma and derangement is termed bioductosis, which causes neuralosis, or chronic stress in the central neural system. This neuralosis reflects on the mind to produce mentosis, or a chronic anxiety syndrome, and concurrently on the body to cause somatosis, or degenerative organic disease.

If the structure of the bioductory system is physically disordered, harm comes to the structure of the central neural system, including the brain, because of this neurophysical coaxiality.

A chronically traumatized bioductory system not only drains the brain of neural capability but also hinders it from receiving normal sustenance and replenishment from a properly functioning soma. Here is the cause of chronic degenerative diseases, including heart attack, cancer, and emotional upset.

The brain, well structured, responds with bell-like clarity to demands. Destructured, from chronic traumatic overburden and undernourishment, it responds erratically and unnaturally.

From the word *Pleneurethic,* three useful terms are derived: *pleneurize, depleneurize,* and *repleneurize.*

Pleneurize means bringing the brain to optimum competence. *Depleneurize* refers to any debilitating process that reduces brain competence. *Repleneurize* alludes to processes by which brain competence may be restored to normal following a period of depleneurization.

Most common causes of harm to the brain are malstructure of mentality and distortions of the bioductory system arrangement. Both destroy the ability of the brain to proliferate normal patterns of energy.

Once the brain is inimically modified, all other tissue systems, including the mind, are pathologically affected according to the pattern of cerebellar distortion.

Pleneurethic aims at cure of chronic disease by correcting the prime source of chronic disturbances to the brain, thereby reversing the course of disease processes. If the brain has been allowed to progress into an irreversibly damaged condition, Pleneurethic is no longer curative. It is, at best, only ameliorative.

Corrective techniques employed by Pleneurethic are: removal of pathological physical trauma on central neurological tissues by physically restructuring anatomical distortion in the bioductory system, and eradication of mental malstructure by assisting the individual to adopt realistic life goals and standards of ethical behavior.

The Pleneurethic approach is structural in physical and mental anatomy and Pleneurethical remedy is primarily aimed at correcting stress-producing structural distortion.

The Pleneurethical appraisal of human affairs is on three levels, each one being separated into three categories. The levels are (1) physical, (2) intellectual, and (3) spiritual (ethical). The three categories are (1) content, (2) structure, and (3) function.

Physical level structures of our body are constructed from material components. Intellectual level structures of the mentality are derived from intelligence and knowledge obtained from our ordinary senses. Spiritual structures are construed from universal ethic.

The idea of *content* is perhaps the easiest category to understand. It is the idea of content and its interrelationship with structure and function that is instrumental in inspiring such healing approaches as medicine and surgery. In medicine we add ingredients to the body, hoping to directly improve its content, beneficially modifying its function and structure. In surgery, we have medicine in reverse. Surgery removes content that has hopelessly deteriorated.

Several disciplines and philosophies believe content to be the only approach to healing. Their adamant refusal to acknowledge a structural approach has imposed hardship upon those who suffer from chronic illness.

Structure is concerned with design and arrangement to produce shape, form, or configuration. Structures are predicated upon meaningful interrelationships between organic parts or stress-bearing members. Proper structure is a prime requisite to content acquisition, utilization, and retention. Proper structure relationship is fundamental to effective and efficient function. If structure fails, both content and function will be jeopardized.

Efforts to save the structure, which through traumatic force has been chronically disorganized, will be unsuccessful if the only avenues of therapy are by way of content replenishment or functional stimulation.

Function is founded on content and structure and is a reflection of the interaction of these two categories. Function is movement and involves manipulation of discrete elements of content within a framework of structure, which itself must be composed of content.

Disorganized function may be precipitated by either structural abnormalities or deviations in content. Structural rearrangement shifts the framework of function and revises the limits of functional activity.

Structure is cause; function is effect.

If we vary the structural cause excessively, we swing the range of function to a new and pathological position in the total spectrum of activity. Functions that are chronically debilitating are synonymous with degenerative operation.

A functional approach to healing chronic illness is not basic, although it may temporarily ease burdensome distress. Important as content and function are in the physical body, structure is the prime factor to be dealt with in successfully and permanently restoring health.

Not only does structure order function and dictate content requirement, but the manner in which a structure is assaulted determines its pattern of collapse. The more complicated the structure, the more complex the symptoms of collapse.

Structural disorders create stresses that, in turn, produce functional abnormalities (mental and physical diseases). Chronic structural disorders of the central neural system elicit chronic diseases. Acute stresses produce acute ailments. Stress that produces excessive structural disorder harmfully alters function and modifies content utilization. Counterstress that corrects structural disorder reverses the disease process and restores the condition for bringing function and content to normal.

Pleneurethic also sees the cause of cerabellar distortions to spring from three primary sources—mechanical, psychological, and chemical.

Mechanical trauma to any sector of the bioductory system produces correlative patterns of chronic physical trauma directly on nerve and brain tissue. This, in turn, affects the structure, function, and content of the brain.

Psychological trauma from mental conflict produces acute patterns of distortion and tension in the brain affecting its working capability.

Chemical trauma from poisons such as alcohol or inadequate amounts of food and liquid may also adversely influence the brain.

Basically, chronic diseases occur in the body because the central neurological resources necessary for health have been chronically impaired after chronic bioductory mishap. Chronic mental problems, in company with chronic physical disease, appear in the form of a chronic anxiety syndrome, especially pronounced when the upper sectors of the bioductory system are damaged.

Since there is an infinite variety of possible patterned distortions in the brain from bioductory trauma, so also is there an infinite variety of patterns of chronic illness—somatic, mental, and emotional.

PART 2

Pleneurethic fills a centuries-old void in man's life which has existed because of the bitter conflict between religion and science. Pleneurethic has none of the abuse to reason presented by mystical church nor the intense, often callous, materialism of uncontrolled science. Pleneurethic forms a common meeting ground for those persons disenchanted with mystical church, and who wish for something more enduring than the flashy novelties that commercial science frequently fetches.

Structure is basic; it provides Pleneurethic with a relevancy and regularity and predictability achieved by no other school. According to Pleneurethical postulate, the brain is the central structure of each individual. The brain is, therefore, the prime target for Pleneurethical philosophy and science and practice.

Interrelationships between essential structures control our life and the way we live it. Important structures over which we have some measure of control are: brain, mentality, body, and the external world with its civilization and culture. In Pleneurethic it is postulated that the Absolute, central engine of the universe, elaborates an animatory force which is available without limit. Hence, it is not a structure to be manipulated by man, nor is it even a matter of any great occupation. It is more pertinent for man to be concerned about his comprehension of those structures over which he exercises some control.

Stresses and tensions are necessary corollaries of organisms in a structured universe. All living structures must bear strain. Too much strain—and the living structure breaks down from overload, and function ceases. Too little strain—and the organism succumbs from disuse and atrophy, or disintegrates as an unaccustomed load is presented it.

In the case of people, incorrect exertion causes structural distortion, and results in functional problems which manifest the signs and symptoms of disease. Also in the case of people, insufficient structural activity leaves them unprepared for emergencies which invariably await them. Such people suffer from immaturity and weakness.

In biological structures, excessive tension from structural distortion inhibits relaxation. Loss of ability to relax, because of chronic structural distortion, breeds chronic disease. Moreover, stresses from several vectors may reinforce one another in the brain to evoke seemingly mysterious, but none-the-less very dangerous, diseases. Such diseases are difficult, virtually impossible, to diagnose or treat unless Pleneurethic principles are understood. Diseases are uniformly misdiagnosed and maltreated if we believe them to be caused by exotic germs, remote reaches of an unconscious sector of mind, or revenge of an incensed Holy Spirit.

For the good of humankind, Pleneurethic strives to simplify and remove mystery from all that which involves biological affairs. Diverse biological events are handily correlated when analyzed in terms of structural distortions, and in terms of transfer of resulting stresses to interrelated organic structures and tissues.

Pleneurethic encompasses all structures and substructures of our world as they impinge upon the brain of humankind individually and collectively. This indeed is a vast expanse, and there are few who see it in its entirety. Most of us must remain content to see only parts of the total pattern, and even then it is difficult to entertain simultaneous comprehension of those few parts we do perceive.

Thinking of structure, we must recognize two broad divisions: macro and micro. Macrostructure is the gross anatomy of any device or object. Macroanatomy considers the basic external shape, and internal main beams which support and absorb major strain in any structural machination. Microstructure, on the other hand, is concerned with the minute particles from which a device or object is constructed. Thus, the microstructure of the human body is composed of cells and noncellular tissues. Some liquids are structural, such as blood with its array of necessary ingredients. The mind is also structured in Pleneurethic as is civilization through its institutions.

Both microstructure and macrostructure are important. But each can be overlooked or overemphasized to the detriment of knowledge. Thus, if we concentrate on microstructure, we see the tree but not the forest. If we become preoccupied with macrostructure, we view the vast reach of the forest, but fail to note its individual trees.

Stress, then, is present in all structures. Normal stresses are present in proper structures. Abnormal strains and stresses occur in distorted structures, to produce many functional problems, which may even reverberate to jeopardize the entire structure.

Signs and symptoms of functional aberration and abnormality, because of structural distortion, run the entire spectrum of mental and physical disease. Efforts of the organism to process or compensate the effects of structural distortion lead to a wide range of pathologies from nightmares and irrational behavior, to ulcers and cancer cell formation.

Pleneurethical therapy relieves undesirable accumulations of distortion in key structures, thereby correcting pathological distortion in correlative structures sympathetically. Improvement in function of biological tissues and organs invariably occurs when pathological distortions in the major and minor structures of the organisms are abated.

Pleneurethic is not a speculative philosophy, nor need it be taken on faith, for it is rooted in the perennially fertile soil of pure science, universal ethic, and absolute law. It is destined to become a major force in the educated world, leading to a more rational and meaningful way of life for every person.

The preceding was extracted from *Pleneurethic,* volume 7, based on postulates and premises enunciated in earlier volumes of Pleneurethical literature.

PART 3

The entire array of Pleneurethical thought and practice is based upon its own concept of the structure and function of the universe. This subject cannot be avoided if one is to establish a rational and realistic way of life and system of therapeutics.

Addressing himself to the tasks of philosophy, Victor Ferkiss states:

> There are three basic questions with which any philosophy . . . must deal: (1) What is man? (2) What is the nature of the universe as it affects man? (3) What is the relationship between man's values and the way in which the universe works? Whether these questions are answered explicitly or implicitly they cannot be ignored. One of the things which separated the great political philosophers such as Plato, Hobbes, and Marx from mere ideologues is that the former deal with these questions directly and attempt to relate subsidiary propositions about the nature of justice to their answers to these basic questions about human nature and destiny.
>
> Unless we know what man is, we have no way of knowing what the possibilities or limits of his actions are, nor can we know what will make him healthy and/or happy.[1]

Pleneurethic comes to grips with these three basic questions, and out of this confrontation is forged a new system of values based on the constructive conservation of neural energy. Universal in scope, its general recognition and acceptance will bring about a healthier and happier existence for all of mankind.

[1]Victor Ferkiss, "Political Philosophy and the Facts of Life," *Zygon,* IX, No. IV (December 1974), p. 272. (University of Chicago Press)

2

THE ABSOLUTE–
CENTRAL ENGINE
OF THE UNIVERSE

PART 1

Pleneurethic conceives as the source of life and the origin of the universe—the Absolute.

Absolute is defined as a pure, dispassionate power from which all emerges. It emits an absolute principle that forms an array of absolute law. This immutable law of the Absolute provides a gantry of force from which such things as mass, motion, dimension, duration, and consciousness are derived.

Here, then, is the immediate basis for our universe and all that is in it.

Nothing can violate absolute law or absolute principle. However, forces within the universe may cancel each other or reinforce each other to our personal advantage or disadvantage. The force of consciousness and animation may ignore forces of material, but only for a time. Water annihilates fire. Fire destroys wood. Fire warms us, cooks our food, or sometimes burns us. Gravity keeps us on the planet or kills us if we fall from sufficient height without a parachute or other saving counterforce invoked in advance. X rays have diagnostic value but will cause cancer and kill us if improperly employed.

Primitive man looked about the earth, experienced an inability to understand or control much of what he saw and, in despair, conjured the image of capricious, revengeful, vindictive gods.

Pleneurethical man looks about and sees the exquisite workings of a flexible and pulsating system, governed by broad parameters but permitting nearly total randominity in minute detail. Even man

13

himself, in some respects, is a minute detail. So, too, are all other animals, plants, clods of earth, water spray, and gases.

Pleneurethic views, as the external giver of life, an animatory force that has been given the name Aramic force.

Aram uses forms fashioned from material to construct a system of life on earth. Aram does not make the environment nor the dust, liquid, or vapor. Aramic force simply uses these components. (I chose this term by adapting basic words and syllables such as RA, MA, and AM which, in combination, produced many words and names of anthropological-metaphysical significance: Rama, incarnation of Vishnu and hero of the Hindu epic; Ramayana, whose name was adopted by many rulers in India and the countries of Southeast Asia influenced by Hindu culture; Amida Buddha; Mara, the tempter of Gautama Buddha; Marae, the ancient sacred places of Polynesia, and many others. Eventually, I arbitrarily settled on Aram as the combination of sounds I was looking for. It exists in Hebrew with the meaning of upland or highland, but its use in Pleneurethic is in line with the definition given above. It should be pronounced ah-ROM.)

The living energy of Aram is endless and inexhaustible. If all life were erased by some cataclysmic cosmic event, Aram would be untouched, unmoved, unmolested.

Aram is not capricious but works patiently in material, according to forces of the universe governing material. Aram cannot override the force controlling physics but must confine itself to physical limitations. *And all life on earth is but Aramification of material in the several life forms we see on land, and in the air, and in the water.*

Aram cares not for any particular physical shape. It presses itself into any viable form whatsoever. If the material environment changes, Aram shifts its expression to another physical form more agreeable to the new environment. Aram is flexible in its choice of material housing.

If Aram is flexible, the Absolute is, by comparison, inflexible.

The Absolute is distant and remote and unapproachable by men.

In Pleneurethic, worship of the Absolute is inappropriate. The Absolute would not find gratification from such worship nor be disposed to confer preferential treatment upon the supplicant. In fact, the Absolute is insensitive to worship by human beings.

For in Pleneurethic there is no deity of limited Christian characteristic. Absolute law is endowed with the power to provide both inanimate dust and the source of animating consciousness called Aram. Absolute moves according to rule. There is no way to contest, argue or plead with either Aram or the Absolute. And indeed, to the believer in the principles of Pleneurethic, there is abiding comfort in the knowledge that the universe is not capricious but orderly.

There is no reassurance in Pleneurethical philosophy for those demanding special dispensation. Neither the Absolute nor Aram can be moved to aid one's friends or destroy one's enemies.

The Absolute abandons no one out of jealousy nor attacks the sinful out of revenge.

The Absolute makes no covenants with any nation or race. Instead, the Absolute is available to all people equally.

Regional morality of provincial gods and superfigures is over-ridden by Pleneurethic's universal concept of the Absolute. If Pleneurethic does violence to regional superfigures around which codifications of morality have been erected, then does it not offset such violence with a viable standard which tends to unify all religions and discourage intersect hatreds?

Pleneurethic is theistic belief based on faith in the rational rather than the mysterious or supernatural.

The term *theism* is used by philosophers and theologians to refer to the idea of a god of superhuman characteristics.

Theism is not a religion but a speculative theory forming a core around which a religion may be constructed. Strict theism, basis for several religions, affirms an Absolute Creator of the universe who also is present in the universe. God thus transcends the universe and is immanent in it. Theists affirm that God not only conceived and constructed the universe but he continues to operate it on a second-by-second basis.

Deists, on the other hand, believe God formed the universe

and all that is in it but withdrew from it once it was created; that he remains detached and separated in a completely supernatural manner. God then, to the deist, is not immanent.

The deists place reason above inspired revelation.

Acosmism is the belief that the universe is separate and distinct from God. Hence, acosmism stands in direct opposition to the pantheistic notion that the universe *is* God.

Pleneurethic is theistic in the sense that it believes there is but one source—the Absolute—which is synonymous with some, but not all, aspects of the theistic concept of God.

It is deistic in the belief that religion should be rational, without mystery; that revelation comes from within the individual and is not restricted to a priestly or clerical class of professional churchmen.

Pleneurethic is acosmistic in that it believes that Absolute is separated from the universe by a series of buffers.

Religion, church dogma, and ethic are not synonymous. Religion is any personally accepted belief that governs behavior; church dogma is a codification of rules prepared by churchmen to foster their worldly church institutional organization; whereas ethic deals with individual conduct that best fosters the needs of the living community, evolution of the species, and the individual's own needs.

The term *religion* was developed from root words which refer to restraint, a holding back, or that which binds from the force of bondage. Basically, religion is a personal commitment to a particular system of beliefs, those beliefs being regarded as inviolable or sacred. The form it assumes is predicated upon one's own convictions developed through contemplation and meditation or a system of rules laid down by others. Religion comes from a desire to believe.

Organized religions proliferate from this willingness to believe.

Few people are inspired to derive their own explanation for the universe, to cultivate their own ethical resources, or seek their own counsel. They prefer to accept (or are harassed into accepting) prefabricated codes of ethics by someone they consider wiser, more forceful, or more experienced spiritually.

Preference is given to principles developed so long ago the principle seems to have been fashioned not from the mind of man but from an oracle resident in ages past. It becomes more credible, more authentic, through association with antiquity.

Organized church religion might well be termed a codification of theological speculation considered to be divinely inspired, designed to control man's behavior for his own good, the good of society, and, in actuality, for the proliferation of the church itself.

Organized religion is potentially powerful. Throughout history it has performed social, economic, political, and military functions. It has, on occasion, not only challenged but taken over, the political power of the state. It has raised and supported armies to carry out strictly church objectives.

Although church religion is basically man-made law, it has not been developed by representatives of the people. Rather, religious codes are dictated by men who arrogate such powers to themselves and who derive their knowledge through alleged inspiration from supernatural sources.

There is nothing in the broad concept of religion that requires a belief in a supernatural power or a god. Religion is simply a firm personal belief in something, a state of mind wherein a set of principles or beliefs is held inviolable.

One need not belong to a church to have a religious attitude. Indeed, any person can entertain a set of beliefs so firmly that these beliefs become a religion to him.

Pleneurethic does not partake of the mantle of a church. It does not interest itself in preparing men's alleged souls for proper presentation of themselves to a godly maker after death. However, Pleneurethic is decidedly concerned with humanism and in easing problems of persons while they are alive on this earth. It deplores departure of the church from its role in the spiritual realm and advent into the realm of undertaking to cure man's physical body.

The Pleneurethicist views the somatic, material portion of our body as having developed on an evolutionary basis. The human body is essentially mechanical on the gross scale. Even on the biochemical level we find atomic chemistry to be perhaps more a study of physics than chemistry, our gross anatomical structure and biochemical function differing little from a lower animal form.

Whether the evolution of the human body from a lower order was at God's wish or command of Buddha principle is not significant to Pleneurethic.

However, Pleneurethic does contend that human beings are more than physical bodies. In addition to this earthly machine constituted from minerals and vapors of this world, we also have a consciousness.

Our human consciousness was not derived from lower forms of life nor was it molded through adaptation of the species. Human consciousness, Pleneurethic believes, was conferred from a common source—aramic force, if you like.

At death, the material body sinks back to its source in the dust, but the consciousness rises to mingle with its source in the heights above. In other words, even though our individual material body is destroyed, the universal living principle, the animatory force we call Aram, which is responsible for all life, never perishes.

Nothing is ever lost in the Pleneurethical universe.

In Pleneurethic we seek to discover the true substance of the law of the universe and to correlate its eternal mandate with the biological capabilities and limitations of the individual.

Man often makes a serious intellectual error in confusing the essence of civil and universal law. He may break civil (man-made) law with impunity or with little consequence. And, so he reasons, he may transgress the forces of the universe with equal avoidance of penalty. But it is the latter whose breach decrees automatic and spontaneous personal discomfort.

It is just as normal to be ill after breach of universal law as it is to be healthy when universal law is scrupulously obeyed.

Pleneurethic is not strictly a religion and it offers no particular method of developing ethical awareness. However, it does believe that the seeds of such awareness or grace are resident within each individual. Each has plenary authority and competency to search his own inner being for contact with the true source of all ethical and philosophical knowledge.

This, then, has been a prime pursuit of Pleneurethic—to determine the eternal (ethical, intellectual, and material) laws of the Absolute and to follow these laws to the best of the individual's ability.

Pleneurethic is not overly concerned with whether an individual believes the universal ethical law to be pronounced by a god of human characteristics, a Buddha-like divine principle, a spirit of Allah, or some other source of divine and eternal power, wisdom, and truth.

Pleneurethic believes there is no essential disagreement between the innermost essence of Christianity, Buddhism, Taoism, Mohammedanism, or Judaism. Details of living forms and conscious awareness techniques may assume limitless variations restricted only by broad specifications decreed by the Absolute.

PART 2

Pleneurethic sees the universe as a system of structures and substructures, all interrelated in varying degrees. Some structures are dominant, others subordinate, and still others alternate their role according to their employment. The Absolute is the prime structure. Life is a fringe structure resulting from various combinations of the forces of material and animative consciousness. These forces stand as a buffer between the Absolute and all life forms on earth. See Fig. 1.

The Absolute of Pleneurethic is seen as emitting an absolute principle which forms an array of absolute law. This immutable law of the Absolute throws a gantry of force from which such things as mass, motion, dimension, and consciousness are derived. Here is the immediate basis for our universe and all that is in it. And here is the source of Pleneurethical truth, because such truth flows from basic structures of the universe.

Material which is apparent to our senses is but the tip of the iceberg. For behind all material that is visible and palpable to our limited range of perception exists an immense amount of invisible material. This is called meta-material in Pleneurethic. That which is true for material is likewise true for consciousness and the animating force of life.

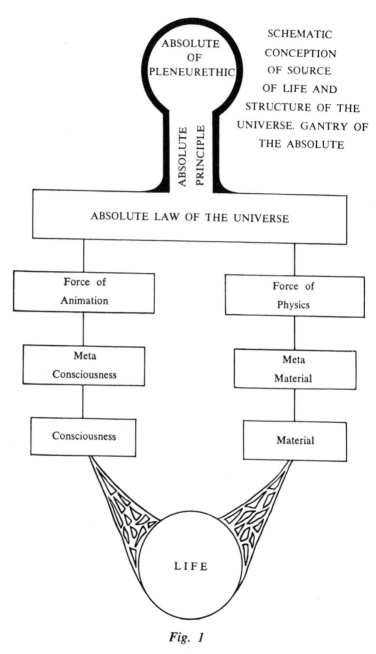

Fig. 1

20

Meta-consciousness is the unseen force of life which resides in a realm beyond our range of perception. This force has been given the name Aramic force.

All life on earth is but the Aramification of material in the several life forms that we see on land and in the air and water.

Aramic force causes life to spring through mineral bodies fashioned from the earth of the world. Such life rises as the steamy fog springs from the sun-drenched watery surface. And as one fog bank envelops another, or a colder fog bank shoulders a warmer fog bank to one side, so will a stronger species eradicate a weaker species—without the slightest reaction from Aram.

Aramic force is the eternal giver of life force. This life force mingles with the clods to form a seething mass of life which writhes, pulses, and surges, each according to its character. The living energy of Aram is endless and inexhaustible, but it must be understood that it is not an entity as such and certainly not a deity, although it has often been mistaken for one.

Since life on earth abides in material physical form, we cannot evade recognition of the laws of physics. For indeed the law of physics is nothing but the absolute law expressed in terms of mass, trajectories, orbits, attractions, repulsions, ducts, levers, transfers, bioelectric coaxial transmission devices, and the like.

To sum up, meta-material is the other end of the continuum which appears as material to our senses. Meta-consciousness is the opposite aspect of the continuum which is sensed as consciousness, animation, and mind. Aram is the arbitrary name given to the dispassionate provider of animatory consciousness (life force) found in all forms of life on earth and elsewhere in the universe.

Stars were struck by the Absolute and sent swirling into space as life took form within that sweep of eternal force. Life takes many forms and each must find its way to useful existence or meaningless death.

Although there is but one way of life prescribed by the Absolute, there are countless styles of living which man may select for his civilization. We identify with the way of the Absolute on earth by adopting a proper life-style and fostering the quality of life in our civilization.

Life-styles which despoil life form, mislead mentality, and degrade the earth from which our material drape is drawn are bad. They are unethical and antagonize the advance of civilization. They are substantially un-Pleneurethical because they contribute little of lasting value to the thrust of life on earth.

All life-styles are good which honor life form, enlighten mentality, and revere its environment. Life-styles which conserve vital capability and foster civilized well-being are good. They are Pleneurethical.

We are better advised to consider the future of civilization than our own status in an obscure hereafter. Civilization is the highest achievement of humankind and as we, ourselves, aid this achievement, so are we blessed in equal proportion.

Pleneurethic sees civilization as the living wheel of majestic dimension which rotates in evolution through space and time to its ultimate destiny.

Pleneurethic's wheel of civilization includes all people and beings of the world. Every individual occupies a position and should assist forward movement of civilization by doing his or her share.

This share should be aimed positively toward good. Overexposure of evil and negative fault-finding argument accomplish little. Continued eradication of bad accomplishes less than progressive expansion of good. For if good is everywhere there will be no place for evil to flourish. But if good is neglected bad will perpetually arise in ever-newer form, as old evil is vacated by a hypercritical evil-oriented society.

It is more relevant to put your shoulder to the wheel of civilization and support its evolutionary advance than to pick up the Cross to stamp out devils, burn witches, or draw and quarter infidels if they refuse conversion to the faith.

The wheel of civilization turns true on the structure of Pleneurethic as we consider what should be done rather than what could be done. For the ethical distance between the possible and the desirable is vast indeed. Simply because something is feasible does not also mean that eternal good will be derived from such an act. We mortals are transient reflections in the clay of absolute principle. Our structural form enables this principle to abide in molecular substance. Individuals shall cleave to that way which resonates with the beat of eternal principle if they would flourish and live abundantly.

The way for civilized life was set by absolute principle. We must take care lest our life-style repudiate the way and lead us to our ruin and that of others about us. Deviation from the way breeds suffering and the loss of real competency.

Blemish which appears on man means his style of life has gone astray from the eternal way. Erasure of all blemish is achieved by the revision of life-styles, a return to the true way. But take care lest the distance of digression exceed the ability of material form to negotiate a complete return.

Attention to the eternal way yields true satisfaction and retention of living form. There is only one structural integrity for health. There are unending numbers of aberrations to mental and physical structure, all of which lead to dissolution of our earthly being and the erosion of civilization.

Universal truth is based upon structure put in place by the Absolute. As we comprehend this structure and align ourselves with it, so we shall be free in equal portion.

The wheel of civilization truly turns on the relevant structural axis formed by the eternal law of Pleneurethic.

Pleneurethic disagrees with any religion which proclaims chronic disease and suffering to emanate from a hostile or vengeful God. Instead, Pleneurethic believes that the basis for total health is a well-structured brain, and that chronic illness comes from chronic brain disability. Chapter 3, therefore, will commence our study of brain from a Pleneurethical point of view. Brain is at the very center of our person; hence, by treating the brain we treat the *entire* person.

3

THE BRAIN–
CENTRAL ENGINE OF MAN

PART 1

Perhaps the easiest way to acquire an initial grasp on Pleneurethic is to consider the brain as a living machine. The brain is structured to fulfil a biological need and functions to produce a biological result. The brain receives input into its structure and functions to transmit output.

The brain is coaxial:

* neuro-chemically with blood which circulates through it to nourish it or poison it;
* neuro-mentally with mind, which manipulates it wisely or unwisely;
* neuro-physically with the external material environment, which protects or injuries it;
* and neuro-socially with other human beings and their cultural institutions.

Therefore, brain and its energy is postulated to be the axial biological reality of life in earth. If brain structure is altered, so that its pattern of operation is modified, this change will be manifested in body tissues and mind and even society, according to the pattern of brain alteration.

Brain stands at the crossroads of our mental and physical being. All things are related to the brain, and in turn the brain relates to all things of its immediate environment. The study and control of these bilateral relationships constitutes the central sphere of Pleneurethic.

Disease is best categorized in terms of the brain and its neural system. Chronic degenerative disease is caused by chronic brain problems which in turn are elicited by chronic bioductory deflections. Acute diseases are from other sources of stress and traumatic disturbance to the brain, except in the case of congenital conditions which are caused by the malformation of the central neural system before birth. Many congenital disorders in children are postulated by Pleneurethic to be due to certain forms of chronic illness in their parents. These parental illnesses are caused by brain conditions inflamed by self-abuse from alcohol, drugs, and the like.

Chronic mental and physical disorders invariably accompany each other because they arise from a common cause—central neural disturbance. Acute illnesses of psychological genesis can also cause dual effects in the mind and the body because of the medical position of the brain. Doctors must be trained to differentiate between the two.

The brain accumulates tension from several sources, both acute and chronic, and reacts according to the aggregate. It must either dissipate this tension through various processes or retain the accumulation and absorb the deleterious consequences.

It is a mistake to believe that the brain is confined to the section of it which resides within the skull. The brain extends down through the spine and makes up what is known as the neural system.

There is no question that the neural system leads the way and regulates the development and operation of other and lesser organic systems of the body. It also influences the way in which the mentality will develop.

We study the development and nature of the brain to achieve perspective and to understand some of the specific forces which exert an influence upon it. We will find that some forces are beneficial and are to be encouraged, other forces are inimical and are to be avoided.

It will be helpful to observe the neural system in its earliest stage of development.

A human brain and peripheral neural system is implicit in

each submicroscopic germ cell. In its submicroscopic stage the brain system (brain, spinal cord and peripheral nerves) is invested with a dual function: to respond to a universal living force and to regulate the development of an individual to be composed of materials available on earth when conditions are propitious for survival.

The submicroscopic neural system in the germ cell will not trigger the developmental unfolding of the germ cell into an individual until certain physical conditions have been met. It would be fruitless for a germ cell to be stimulated out of its relative inert state into a stage of development if suitable materials were unavailable from which a material body could be constituted.

Perhaps two examples will illustrate the point involved.

The first example will use the plant germ cell (seed). Simple as a vegetable is, certain conditions must prevail before it can survive. Before the primitive regulatory system of a vegetable seed will initiate the developmental process, certain environmental factors must be obtained. Thus, the temperature of the seed must be within a certain range. If freezing weather conditions exist, the seed's regulatory system will not trigger the development and material acquisition process. In addition to proper temperature environment there must be suitable amounts of moisture available. Finally, the plant seed must be in earth of proper consistency, being neither too hard nor too soft, containing adequate amounts of finely divided minerals of suitable dimension.

If all of the environmental requirements are properly met, the seed will be triggered and commence to gather material to itself and an individual of the plant kingdom will be formed.

Simple as this process is, there is a chance for the plant's regulatory system to trigger development before all survival conditions have been met. Thus, it is possible for a seed lying on the floor of a damp, dark, warm cellar to be triggered out of its inert state. However, since material in the form of minerals is unavailable to the seed because of the hard-packed earthen floor of the cellar, the plant seed may simply rot away and eventually become a part of the dirt of the cellar floor.

Although plants do not have an extensive regulatory system as the brain system in a human being, they have one nevertheless. Plants are not called up for the variety of behavior that is expected from human beings. They do not have the capability for running, dancing, fighting, singing, writing books, or making love. They are expected to remain rooted in one spot, grow larger and produce more seed. A very primitive regulatory system is all that is required to control the development of a vegetable.

Our second example will deal with the developmental process of the human seed as contrasted to the development of a vegetable seed. As we have already seen in the case of the vegetable only one seed is needed to produce an individual if all environmental factors are satisfactory. Because of the automatic nature of the vegetable seed, there is a good chance that it will emerge prematurely from the inert stage, and perish because all necessary environmental prerequisites have not been fully met. In the case of the human individual two seeds are ordinarily required. The requirement for the union of two seeds to produce a human individual introduces additional significant guarantees of successful survival over and above those enjoyed by the unilateral action of a vegetable seed.

Disregarding the process of parthenogenesis, each human being commences with the union of two microscopic organisms. One type of organism is of receptive nature and descends serenely at maturity from its birthplace in the ovary to its seat of prospective developmental activity within the uterus. The other type of organism is supplied by the millions during copulation. These other organisms are aggressive by nature and feverishly seek to penetrate to the very core of the cell which was designed to receive their advance.

Nature endeavors to improve the chances of human seed survival by requiring that both hosts of the parent germ cells be alive and reasonably healthy at the time of conception. Contrast this with the vegetable whose ancestors may have been dead for years before the inert seed finds a haven presenting development possibilities.

Further safeguards are introduced. The receptive human

germ cell cannot mature unless a female human being has been able to survive in a suitable environment for about twelve years or more. This is the first safeguard insuring the egg when fertilized will be met with a favorable geographical environment.

Not only must the female have survived the environment but the female must be in proper age bracket and in suitable health. If the female is too young or too old or too sick to properly care for the offspring, the chances are that no germ cells will be produced. Moreover, since the physical movement of any female is more or less hindered during the latter stages of pregnancy she does not ordinarily submit wantonly to male advances, but only after a display of love, affection and competency has assured her that she will be taken care of during the critical period ahead. There must be fulfilment of a love and affection requirement in addition to a good geographical climate.

A final safeguard against the triggering of the development of a human egg (germ cell) is that it must await the presence of another germ cell produced by a second human being of male character which has not only been able to survive the existing environment for a period of years, but has also been able to convince the female of his ability to care for her and their progeny.

There are more safeguards, but to enumerate them would belabor the point. They pertain to a host of internal and external requirements of biological, sociological, and spiritual nature.

It is palpably evident that the triggering mechanism in the human germ cell will not commence operations until a vast amount of preliminary activity has successfully transpired. When the submicroscopic neural system in the human germ cell finally commences its task of directing and regulating the development of another individual, there is a fairly good chance that the venture will be successful. At least the chances for success are greater than in the case of the vegetable seed.

So from the very beginning we discover that the submicroscopic neural system has certain capabilities, limitations, and requirements in order for it to survive and to successfully supervise the development of an individual. Even in the preliminary stage preceding the germ disk stage it has required: a supply of material food upon which to feed, proper temperature of the surrounding material, and sufficient fluid to act as a vehicle for the transportation of material from which the individual is to be composed. Moreover, notwithstanding the possibility of a few children as a result of rape, a certain degree of approval, affection, receptive willingness, and *demonstrated competency* must prevail before a hardy race of people can be generated. This is particularly true in the colder and more vigorous climates. A superior race of people cannot and never will be built on the basis of lechery, prostitution, and a welfare state. It can only be built on capability for love, affection, approval, mutual regard, integrity, and confidence in the ability of the other. Such is the stuff of great nations.

We return our attention to the development of the embryonic neural system.

The human embryo, which contains the all-important neural system, is formed from the union of an ovum and a spermatazoa. After the two nuclei of these individuals have united, a single individual nucleus is formed which begins to divide and redivide. The cells formed by division from the original fertilized ovum are independent and shift their position with respect to each other. They are distinct individual cells and have not yet settled down into a fixed tissue relationship with other neighboring cells in the morula. At this stage they remain within the confines of a membrane called the zona pellucida. As the zona pellucida vanishes the cells settle down into a hollow spherical relationship which is called a blastocyst. As few as 60 cells may form a blastocyst of which 55 may serve as food for the other 5 cells which are destined to form an embryo and later a fetus. The embryonic area of the blastocyst shows no differentiation in its earliest stages. One of the first features of the embryonic cellular mass is the formation of the primitive streak. This streak is simply a line of cells which have developed an opacity in the embryonic tissue because they are multiplying at a faster rate and thereby contrast with neighboring cells which are not developing at such a furious rate. The primitive streak, the first identifiable cellular differentiation in the embryonic tissue, will become the spinal system. The opacity of the primitive streak implies that the cells which constitute the primitive streak are growing at a much more rapid rate than the surrounding tissues which will later become muscles, etc. There is no question that there is intensive cell growth and feverish cellular activity along the line of the primitive streak.

The first division of the fertilized ovum creates two individual cells called blastomeres. These blastomeres continue to divide, forming a hollow cellular sphere called a morula within the confines of a limiting membrane, the zona pellucida. As the zona pellucida disappears and the morula is filled with fluid it becomes a blastocyst about the fifth day after fertilization. The earliest identifiable tissue within the blastocyst, at around the twelfth day after inception, is a rapidly growing mesoderm and a more rapidly growing and larger germ disk called the ectodermal plate. It is from the mesoderm that the bones, muscles, and connective tissues of our body are formed. The ectoderm will divide into the neurectoderm and skin ectoderm to form the nerve system, brain, and skin. The mesoderm tissues grow slower than the ectoderm but the fastest growing portion of the mesoderm compares with the dorsal lip of the blastopore, which becomes the vertebral column and forms the nerviducts.

Crosssectional pictures of a human fertilized ovum of around thirteen days show the germ disk to be the largest portion of the formative cell section. Of course the yolk sack is larger than the germ disk or ectoderm but the yolk sack is composed of nourishing material which will be consumed by the developing ectoderm, mesoderm, and entodermal tissues. The yolk sack is not composed of totipotential formative cells but consists of supporting cells to be sacrificed as a temporary source of food for the embryo. The yolk sack tides the formative cells over until they can establish an operational system capable of deriving sustenance from the walls of the uterus.

Our neural system commences as a hollow sphere of ectodermal cells. This sphere joins another group of entodermal cells. Extending from the line of fusion or primitive streak we find the neural plate which is the site of intense cellular activity. At the end of the third week the neural groove is completed. The embryo is hardly more than one-sixth of an inch long at this juncture. With the passing of the fourth week the neural tube is closed and the shape of the brain, spinal cord, and nerves both cranial and spinal are beginning to assume the same distinctive shape which will exist in maturity. The neural system in the early weeks of development shows clear and distinct differentiation whereas the embryonic tissues which are developed into other organs and tissues of the body are barely identifiable, with the exception of our skin, and a very rudimentary vascular system.

All thinking persons are astonished when they witness the rapidity with which the brain system is established in the embryo. It is well worth contemplating the great significance of this early sharp differentiation of the neural cells. They do not arrange themselves haphazardly, but are organized according to plan. This plan, according to Pleneurethic, is associated with the animatory forces. It just does not happen as a fortuitous event on our earthly level, although it may be observed as a random event from the cosmic level.

If the neural cells constituting the brain fail to shift themselves into proper position, our brain would fail to form properly. It is well worth considering the force which causes these individual primitive cells to move and join with other cells in just the correct pattern. In the beginning of the formation of the human embryo, the formative cells are free to shift and change their position at will by their ameboid movement capability.

The formation of the circulatory system of the embryo, together with heart and liver, follows close and hard upon formation of the brain system. However, the heart and liver do not assume their distinctive and mature identifiable shape as soon as the brain system.

In our original work we postulated that the capillary network was the most highly specialized and important part of the vascular system because it was the part which split the flow of blood into venous blood and lymphatic fluid.

This assertion is supported by the work of embryologists which demonstrates that, in the embryo, the capillaries and aorta are the first portions of the circulatory system to be established in the embryo. After the capillary network is well developed, portions of the network enlarge to connect with the aorta. Other large arteries develop separately but only after the capillary network has been built.

The brain system is capable of emerging from a submicroscopic point in a germ cell into an organ weighing upward of eight pounds in an average human being, and at the same time controlling other areas in the germ cell which unfold to become bone, muscle, or connective tissue.

All cells in our body enjoy the capability of reproducing themselves except our nerve cells. Bone cells, and some other cells in our body reproduce themselves through a direct division process called amitosis. In amitosis the nucleus of the cell simply constricts in the middle and then separates forming two nuclei and two cells within a very short time. Muscle cells, connective tissue cells, etc., reproduce themselves indirectly through a complex process called mitosis which may require a few hours to complete. Basically the process of mitosis is a complex division of components of the nucleus followed by cleavage of the cytoplasm to form two cells from the original parent.

Nerve cells do not possess the capability of dividing or reproducing themselves in any way. The lack of capacity for nerve cell reproduction in the same individual precludes eternal life of a physical or material nature.

As nerve cell bodies perish they are never replaced through mitosis or amitosis. However, I hasten to add that cutting of nerve cell processes or tracts does not necessarily or ordinarily kill the nerve cell body. It is possible for a severed neural axonic process to regrow to its original length in somewhat the same manner that it originally extended itself as bone, muscle, and connective tissues proliferated under its control.

The singular fact that the human nerve cell is the only type of cell in our body incapable of reproducing itself by division is of special significance. A statement of the full array of implications on this point will not be essayed at this juncture.

Embryologists do not agree upon the proliferation of the original microscopic brain and peripheral neural system. Some maintain that axonic processes extend themselves from their nerve cell body in the microscopic brain through interstices of cellular tissues finally arriving at the destination where their effectors are located.

Other embryologists proclaim that nerve cell bodies are connected by nerve tracts to their effectors (muscles, etc.) from the very beginning. This second contention, which seems the most logical, follows Pleneurethical view and enjoys our support and endorsement.

The original totipotential cell creates the formative mass of cells in the morula, as contrasted to the second group of cells which will produce both a protective membrane of cells and a yolk to nourish the embryo. The totipotential cells split into ectoderm, entoderm, and mesoderm. The neurectoderm cells retain communication with the skin ectodermal cells, the entodermal, and mesodermal cells by means of embryonic nerve tracts. As the embryo unfolds, the nerve tracts extend to permit expansion of the embryonic mass, thereby retaining the integrity of neural communications.

It is interesting to note some of the principles of growth of secondary nerve processes which arise to support the primary neural system which was present from the very beginning. In the beginning of the embryonic stage, the primary matrix of the neural system is laid down along with more primitive entodermal and mesodermal cell tissues. The secondary budding nerve processes, which emerge as stubs from the nerve cell body, develop ameboidlike tips. These tips create feelers which determine the detailed course of the nerve tract as it intimately follows the course of the original nerve tracts, blood vessels, or other nerve fibers which have previously made the journey and directed the growth of the embryo into a fully developed fetus. These projecting tips follow a detailed and tortuous course through intercellular spaces within the tissue being penetrated by the nerve as it traces the course of the primary nerve.

We can learn much from studying reconstructed drawings

of microscopic studies of human embryos in very early stages of development. There are many examples of such work. Perhaps an average example might be similar to the one presented on page 129 of the thirty-second edition of *Gray's Anatomy*. In this illustration of a human embryo less than one-half inch long, the spinal and cranial nerves are shown in remarkably distinct clarity, and have developed into nearly the identical configuration which is observable in full maturity of a human individual. However, in this same embryo such things as the mouth, arms, legs, etc. do not resemble those of a human being, or anything else as a matter of fact, except perhaps a marine monster.

So, in an embryo less than one-half inch long, the shape of the brain system is unbelievably well developed and resembles with great fidelity its future configuration, while the shape of other organs and appendages are very rudimentary and indistinct indeed. There is much room for serious contemplation here.

In the very beginning we can expect that the primary nerve cells are connected directly by embryonic nerve tracts to the somatic cells which will later through division and redivision become muscles, bones, connective tissue, skin, and the like. Thus, nerve cell bodies and nerve tracts are connected to their destination and are in complete existence from the inception of the embryo. As subsequent secondary nerve cells are formed they extend their processes following along the course laid down by the original nerve tracts from that particular nerve cell section of the brain.

In the reconstructed drawing just mentioned, the volume of the space occupied by the brain, spine, and peripheral nerves appeared to represent about 75 percent of the space occupied by the entire embryo. This should not seem astonishing at all. It is a well-known fact that at birth the brain alone is about one-quarter of its adult size. At the end of the first year of life the brain has reached nearly 75 percent of its adult size. It is evident from these rough statistics that the neural system in the human embryo and early childhood grows much faster during the first few years of life than any bone or muscle system of our body. Indeed, the neural system enjoys the most rapid development of any tissue system of the body. It is fully operational at an age when the infant's arms and legs are flabby pieces of nearly useless material.

Of even greater interest are such illustrations as the one of a human embryo about one-quarter inch long in the fifth week of development, appearing on page 189 of the thirty-second edition of *Gray's Anatomy*. Here again the spinal nerve assembly and the cranial nerves stand out in great detail. At this stage of somatic development arms and legs are not identifiable. The mouth and ears do not appear as such and visceral organs are hardly identifiable. Yet such objects as the trigeminal nerve ganglion of the fifth cranial nerve in the head stand out clearly and in exactly the same shape that it will be a few years later when it reaches its full size.

There is no question that the brain system leads the way and regulates the development and operation of other and lesser organic systems of the body. At this stage, mentioned above, hardly any arteries are formed except for the arteries which will carry blood to the central nervous system.

In the earliest stages of embryonic development the location of the embryonic effector mechanism, and the location of the primary cell body section of the brain are quite close. As the embryo grows larger, the distance between the primary cell body and its effector organ increases. As the distance increases, the axonic connection between the two must also extend itself to maintain the original connection. This ability of cell body axons to increase their length has been proven in experiments by able embryologists. In these experiments embryonic nerve cells were placed in a culture favorable to their survival and growth. As the nerve cells grew larger, the axonic processes extended themselves, even in the absence of other cells.

It appears that from the very beginning the brain system is the chief ingredient of the human being, and all other organs or appendages are simply devices to support the survival of the brain system. Since the cells in the neural system are incapable of reproducing themselves in any particular individual, the only way to perpetuate the brain system is to create new individuals as progeny of the original individuals. A dual system of matching and interlocking germ cells is utilized for this purpose.

Embryologists have provided us with much useful information pointing up the leading role played by the brain system in the development of the human being. In the earliest stages of embryonic development we find the brain system to be the one which develops first and in greatest identifiable detail. For example, study of the development of the skull of the embryo indicates that the cranial nerves and spinal cord are formed long before the skull bones begin to ossify. After the neural system is laid down cartilage is formed in a chondrification process and surrounds the nerves to construct an embryonic foramen for their passage. The nerve tracts are established first, and later protective osseous tissues join and fuse with each other forming a hole in the skull through which the preexisting cranial nerves now pass. The same process holds true for that master gland, the hypophysis or pituitary, which, composed of half gland and half nerve tissue, hangs by a short infundibulum from the base of the brain. The hypophysis is cradled in a bony nest called the sella turcica of the sphenoid. This bony nest forms long after the hypophysis is identifiable and operative. To put it the other way around, the hypophysis is plainly identifiable a few short weeks after the embryo has commenced to form after conception occurs. The sella turcica requires months to take its shape in cartilage, and additional months are required for transformation of the chondrification into osseous tissue.

The axons with their terminal end fibers which bridge the ever-increasing distance between controlling nerve cell bodies in the brain and effector organs are essential in the development of our human organization. Reliable communication is one of the first and most important devices which is established in any organization involving more than one individual.

Nerve tracts transmit neural messages at varying speeds depending upon the size of the nerve tract. The velocity of neural impulses also changes with the type of nerve involved. Nerve tracts which have a lipid covering are said to be myelinated or medullated. The velocity of a nerve impulse along a large-caliber myelinated nerve in the central nervous system can reach 120 meters per second. The velocity at which a message travels along a small-diameter medullated nerve in the central nervous system may be as low as 5 meters per second. Myelinated nerve fibers located in the peripheral nervous system may conduct impulses at a rate between 3 and 15 meters per second. Unmedullated nerve fibres without a lipid covering transmit impulses at a rate between 0.5 and 2 meters per second.

It is clear that neural messages are not of a totally electrical nature, otherwise the speed would be greater. However, researchers agree that the neural impulse is part electrical and part chemical.

Medullated nerve fibers are colored white due to the lipid covering. These medullated or myelinated fibers are found in the white matter of the brain, and spinal cord. They also constitute the greater part of our cranial and spinal nerves.

The myelin, or fatty covering, serves to insulate and protect the nerve tract which it invests, and also serves as a nutritional reserve to sustain the nerve during periods of short nutritional supply. The myelin coating is not harmed by water, but alcohol dissolves the coating and leaves the nerve unprotected. A nerve demyelinated through excessive consumption of alcohol becomes hypersensitive and undernourished, followed by eventual collapse.

Nerve tissues which are gray are invested with less lipid covering than the white nerve tissue. Gray neural tissue is found in the brain, and in smaller amounts in the ganglia. The ganglia of course are small nerve cell concentrations located in the peripheral portion of our nervous system and act as relay stations to connect nerve tracts together so that greater distances and tissue areas may be traversed. Basically the gray matter is composed of nerve cell bodies, and the white matter constitutes the nerve tracts. Some tracts are more heavily endowed with white lipid covering than other tracts, making them whiter or grayer in comparison.

The oily lipid covering which invests our nerve tracts is there for a reason and if it is removed we may expect to suffer some consequences. The oily lipid covering reduces the coefficient of friction as the nerve tract glides through nerviducts as the body flexes and extends. Without this oily coating nerve tracts may not move easily in shifting nerviducts and inside the neurolemma and endoneurium.

The more closely packed the nerve tracts the greater the amount of white lipid covering. This is especially apparent in the brain and spinal cord, where large and important concentrations of nerve tracts occur. If the fatty covering of the nerve tracts is removed we may expect grave problems to occur. Oil is one of the leading insulators against loss of electrical charge. Almost all electrical circuit breakers which handle quantities of electrical power are filled with oil. So are all large fixed electrical capacitors and heavy transformers filled with oil.

Can you imagine what havoc would occur in our brain and spinal cord if much of the oily insulating material from the discrete nerve tracts was dissolved away by excessive and prolonged consumption of alcohol or cutting acids of certain fruits? One nerve tract would be grounded to another nerve tract, and communications between separate nerve cell sections in the brain would be disrupted or distorted. Many years may be required for the excessive consumption of these alcoholic beverages to work their violence, but the destruction is eventually accomplished and a human derelict is formed.

Nerve cell bodies are capable of receiving stimulatory impulses from sensitive receptors located at the end of those nerve tracts which emanate from cell bodies. The processes or tracts which connect the sensory nerve ending to the nerve cell body are called dendrites. These dendrites may be equipped with a great variety of receptor organs. Dendrite receptor endings are sensitive to vibration. These vibrations, depending upon the type of receptor end organ, may be interpreted by the cell body as heat, cold, sight, hearing, position of body appendages, pleasant pressure, painful pressure, psychic messages, extrasensory perception, and traffic from what is often referred to as the divine.

The simplest type of receptor is nothing but the raw end of a dendrite which has been deprived of any lipid covering whatsoever. Pain receptors are dendrites free of any covering at their free terminal. Special receptor organs are required at the terminal end of dendrites to respond to heat, cold, and various types of pressure. Other types of receptor organs are required to provide us with a proprioceptive sense of the location of such appendages as arms and legs. A final specialized receptor organ is required to intermediate between dendrite terminals and vibrations of life force and other intelligences from the divine.

A point to remember is that receptor organs are composed of tissue. Should this tissue be deprived of normal blood supply and brain regulation, the sensitivity and fidelity of our nerve receptors may be seriously impaired.

The width of the band of vibration in the vibratory spectrum to which our sensory receptors are receptive is severely limited. For this reason we are unaware of a vast multitude of vibrations which are occurring unnoticed by our consciousness. For example, our auditory apparatus is sensitive to a range of vibrations between approximately 16 cycles per second to about 20,000 cycles per second in the average human being. We are unaware of vibrations lower than about 16 cycles per second or beyond 20,000 cycles per second. Thus, our auditory equipment is capable of appreciating an audio frequency band of only about 19,984 cycles per second. This is a very narrow band of vibrations in the vast expanse of the vibratory spectrum.

The same thing is true with our eyes as with our ears. Our visual equipment is capable of detecting only a relatively narrow band of vibratory wavelengths. The average person cannot respond visually to wavelengths longer than that of infrared waves or shorter than ultraviolet waves.

That which is true of our senses of sight and hearing is also true of our other senses. Our senses of smell, taste, touch, and body position are severely attenuated and respond to a very small range of stimuli actually present in our environment. For example, our sense of touch is so limited that we cannot even feel still air about us, let alone distinguish between oxygen, hydrogen, or carbon monoxide gases by our sense of touch. Also our sense of touch is so limited and feeble that it cannot feel into the interior of such objects as rocks or steel bars to locate hard or soft spots in the consistency of those materials.

Our idea of material objects and the world we live in would be totally different if we had a more sensitive or stronger group of sensory organs. Our present conception of the characteristics of material would also be vastly modified if our senses were responsive to a greater expanse of the vibratory spectrum.

If our senses were more sensitive, stronger, and capable of wider frequency response, we might feel that there was no material in the world at all. Or, perhaps, we might believe that there was a great deal more material about us than seems to exist as determined by our present complement of sensory apparatus.

Ontological changes in the intrauterine development of a human embryo clearly trace the evolutionary history or phylogeny of a family of living individuals in which the human being is the most advanced member.

As one observes the transformation of a fertilized ovum through embryonic stages to become a fetus, it is startling to note that at one time the embryo has distinct gill slits similar to some oceanic creature. In the beginning the embryo looks as if it is destined to be a fish, and a few weeks later, after traversing the marine period, it looks as if it might be headed toward some lower vertebrate creature such as a hog. However, if all goes well about nine months later that which emerges is surely identifiable as a human being.

As all this metamorphosis is occurring, we note that the system which develops first and controls the process is the system which changes the least after the first few months of fetal life: the brain system.

Intrauterine unfolding of the brain system of man is especially faithful in traversing nearly identical cellular differentiation as traced by animal individuals in lower vertebrate species. The brain system of man is very similar to that of a pig in the early embryonic stages.

Although man is intellectually superior to the pig, our neural evolutionary lineage is based directly upon the evolution of the swine, and other preceding and succeeding types.

It is through the use of our brain capability developed in later stages of our phylogenic history that we are able to separate ourselves ethically, morally, and intellectually from lower animals.

It should be clearly understood that although we may not be direct descendents of fish, swine, and later the monkeys, we are indebted to them for our basic anatomical structure and physiological function. A vast amount of work was expended in developing the basic anatomical design of the vertebrate group of living organisms. A massive development program was involved in establishing a successful and efficient program of functional interrelationships among the several organic systems of, say, the fish and monkey. The somatic portion of the human being is based upon nearly identical anatomical and functional design as that to be found in the lower forms of animal life. We may not have descended from them through variations of their seed, but definite use was made of knowledge derived from designing the monkey in producing the more advanced design model of the human being.

We now turn our attention to the division and operation of the human brain.

The brain of man is composed of three distinct sections—the hind brain (rhombencephalon), which is attached immediately to the upper end of the spinal cord; the mid brain (mesencephalon); and the fore brain (prosencephalon).

The hind brain includes the medulla oblongata, the pons, and the cerebellum. There is a cavity within the hind brain filled with fluid. This cavity is called the fourth ventricle by anatomists. Eight of the twelve cranial nerves emerge from the surface of the hind brain. One of these nerves is the vagus which travels to all visceral organs such as: heart, lungs, gastrointestinal tract, liver, etc. The vagus constitutes a large part of the parasympathetic segment of the peripheral nervous system. Other nerves which spring from the hind brain's surface are those which proceed to the head and neck tissues.

The hind brain contains nerve cell centers which control the heart and breathing apparatus, the gastrointestinal canal, and all organs secreting juices into the canal. The hind brain nerve cell sections together with their axonic extensions seem to be responsible for internal housekeeping affairs. Here is the seat of the infraconciousness.

The hind brain was the first of our brains to develop in the early historical stages of our phylogeny. The hind brain directs internal operations on a level below our ordinary consciousness. We are not aware of the vast multitude of internal tasks which it is closely directing second by second throughout our lifetime.

Not only does the hind brain throw connecting fibers to our viscera, but it also issues nerve tracts which connect it with other portions of the brain. This is necessary for coordination between the various sections of the brain.

The cerebellum seems to be the part of our hind brain which provides for refinement of coordination of body movement. A cerebellum which is not functioning properly permits varying degrees of body discoordination—people whose cerebellums are not functioning well cannot walk properly nor can they execute precise movements of their hands and arms.

The floor or anterior wall of the fourth ventricle is a famous place for anatomists. The floor of the fourth ventricle is formed by the posterior surfaces of the pons and the inner open part of the medulla oblongata. It is from the floor of the fourth ventricle in the hind brain that we find the nerve cell source of origin for many of the cranial nerve tracts. If the blood supply to the nerve cells forming the floor of the fourth ventricle is reduced, we may logically anticipate an impairment in the action of the cranial nerves arising from that section.

The pons consists of nerve tracts which connect the hemispheres of the cerebellum. The pons also joins the mid brain above with the medulla oblongata below. The nerve cell centers for the fifth, sixth, seventh, and eighth cranial nerves are located in the pons. The mesencephalon, or mid brain, is a very short section of the brain stem. It contains the aqueduct of Sylviys, which connects the fourth ventricle in the hind brain with the third ventricle located in the fore brain. The mid brain contains many nerve tracts connecting various sections of the brain with each other. It also contains nerve tracts which pass between the spinal cord and the fore brain. The mid brain is noteworthy because of the third and fourth cranial nerves which arise from its interior.

The fore brain, or prosencephalon, is the largest of the three sections of the brain. The fore brain is divided by anatomists for convenience of study into the telecephalon and the diencephalon. The telecephalon, or cerebrum, is the largest part of the brain. The cerebrum is divided into two cerebral hemispheres, each hemisphere containing a ventricle filled with fluid. The two cerebral hemispheres of the cerebrum are connected by the diencephalon formation. This formation encloses the third ventricle which is also filled with fluid and is a part of the diencephalon.

Although the diencephalon is of smaller volume than the telencephalon or cerebrum, it contains many extremely important nerve tissue structures. Two very interesting parts of the diencephalon are the large masses called the thalami. The thalami are formed by an enormous thickening process from a portion of the embryonic neural system known as the neural tube. The thalami are the largest and most important parts of the diencephalon. The thalamus is the most important organ for correlating sensory impressions in primitive vertebrates. However, in man, other centers occupy a higher position in sensory interpretation. In lower vertebrate forms, such as the reptile, the diencephalon forms an epiphysis which develops into a parietal eye. In man, the parietal eye is identifiable in the human embryo, but it does not develop into a mature human parietal eye as in the case of the reptile.

Phylogenically speaking, the oldest portion of the thalamus is termed the palaeothalamus. The newest portion of the thalamus, having reached its greatest development in monkeys and man, is termed the neothalamus.

The thalamus has a variety of functions. It contains nerve tracts which connect many parts of the brain and co-ordinates some activities. The thalamus can itself experience such sensations as pain, permitting finer discriminations to occur in more advanced areas of the telecephalon.

Within the thalamus we find the laterial geniculate body, pulvinar, and superior colliculus, all of which are associated with the lower visual activities. Anatomically speaking, the hypothalamus includes the floor of the third ventricle, the hypophysis and its infundibulum, the optic chiasma, and the subthalamic tissues, etc. The hypothalamus is a very important part of the diencephalon. Portions of the hypothalamus contain nerve cell centers associated with regulating our viscera on the autonomic or infraconscious level.

Here is the seat of control for such organs as the heart, liver, stomach, intestines, blood vessels, etc. If the nerve cell tissues in the hypothalamus are deprived of their normal blood supply, many frightening irregularities may occur in the function of our visceral organs.

Primitive vertebrate creatures depend upon the palaeothalamus for interpretation of harmful or beneficial stimuli. The palaeo‑ thalamus has been replaced by higher appreciative centers in man.

However, the Pleneurethicist believes that these lower sensory centers react to such harmful stimuli as adverse neural pressure along nerve tracts. The sensation recorded by these lower centers is that of worry and an all-pervasive feeling of anxiety and apprehension. Conversely, freedom from harmful neural pressures or strain causes a feeling of irrepressible well-being and zest for life to be registered in these lower interpretive centers. The parasympathetic neural control center springs from nerve cells situated in the anterior part of the hypothalamus, whereas the sympathetic center arises from nerve cell bodies located in the posterior portion of the hypothalamus. Nerve cell tracts from the anterior and posterior portions of the hypothalamus travel divergent courses to their final destination in our viscera. Thus, the sympathetic nerve tracts proceed down the spinal cord and issue as spinal nerves in what is called the thoraco lumbar outflow. Part of the parasympathetic outflow travels as fibers comprising some of our cranial nerves, the most important one being the vagus nerve. The other part of the parasympathetic nerve system proceeds from its control center in the hypothalamus, down the spinal cord, and out by way of spinal nerves in the socral region.

As we have learned, the sympathetic and parasympathetic nerves operate antagonistically but in a coordinated way to control such things as: sleep rhythm, sexual activities, heat regulation, fat, and carbohydrate metabolism. Thus the hypothalamus controls the very basic functions of our body.

The hypothalamus also contains considerable tissue involved in eyesight. The optic chiasma picks up visual activity from the eyeball and optic nerve which penetrate the optic chiasma. From the optic chiasma fibers proceed through the optic tract and continue on through the tuber cinereum, past the cerebral peduncle, to the laterial geniculate body, past the pulvinar and to the superior colliculus. The lateral geniculate body contains nerve cells which relay optic impressions through the optic radiation to reach the higher visual interpretive centers. These centers are located in the cortex of the occipital lobe of the cerebrum or telencephalon. There is a tremendous amount of neural anatomy connected with sight. If the neural cells and tracts do not receive proper blood supply from the internal carotid vertebral arteries, and other cerebral arteries, our visual sensitivity may indeed deteriorate. The amount of blood flowing through these arteries is regulated by nerve cell control centers probably located in the diencephalon.

The hypophysis is of striking appearance and is an inestimably important part of the diencephalon. The hypophysis is half gland and half nerve and hangs from the floor of the diencephalon. The posterior portion of the hypophysis is the neural part and contains a cavity which is continuous with that of the third ventricle. The posterior lobe of the hypophysis does not contain nerve cells. It does contain nerve fiber endings of tracts which originate from nerve cell bodies in the diencephalon.

It seems clear, therefore, that the glandular portion of the hypophysis is under direct control of nerve cell bodies in the diencephalon. The hypophysis is highly vascular and contains a very rich supply of blood capillaries necessary to supply the relatively heavy requirements of that organ. The glandular portion of the hypophysis of course secretes a master fluid which has profound regulatory effect upon the operation of all other glands in the body. This effect is both direct in the case of some subordinate glands such as the thyroid, and indirect in the case of other glands.

The hypophysis receives its blood supply from the internal carotid artery by way of the branching superior and inferior hypophyseal arteries. The nerve center which controls the state of vasodilation or vasoconstriction of these arteries is probably situated in the diencephalon, with perhaps influence from higher centers in the telencephalon.

The telencephalon, a part of the prosencephalon, contains basically the cerebral hemispheres and their ventricular cavities. It also includes a small portion of the front portion of the hypothalamus and third ventricle. Each cerebral hemisphere contains an outer convoluted gray covering consisting mainly of nerve cell bodies and abundant networks of blood capillaries, arterioles, and arteries. The outer gray covering is called the cerebral cortex. The inner portion of the cerebral hemispheres contains a white substance which consists of billions upon billions of nerve tracts which connect the nerve cell bodies in the cortex with various destinations. These destinations can be such places as: other nerve cell centers in the brain, or the peripheral neural tract system by way of the cranial nerves or by way of the spinal cord and spinal nerve roots.

A lifetime could be devoted to a study of the cerebrum. The cerebrum contains the higher centers of sensation, appreciation, and fine discrimination of events brought to its attention. Nerve cell centers in the cerebrum control movements of our arms, legs, facial muscles, and speech mechanisms, etc. It is here that impressions are registered as sight, hearing, taste, smell, etc. The cerebrum is the center for the development of conditioned reflexes, and habitual responses. Memory, judgment, and other abstract operations are conducted by nerve cell sections of the cerebrum.

The front area of the cerebrum has been called the silent area of the brain because damage to that area does not seem to precipitate constitutional or specific symptoms. It is felt by anatomists and physiologists that this area exerts a general steadying tendency on behavior. Feelings of well-being or vague feelings of unpleasantness are generally accepted as being generated by the frontal area of the telencephalon as well as in the hypothalamus. It determines in part the personal reaction to frustration or pleasant events. Damage to nerve cells in this area of the brain definitely results in character changes, reduction in power of concentration, limiting of span of attention, and increased emotional instability.

It is a well-known fact that sham rage is demonstrated when nerve tracts are severed between the frontal cortex of the telencephalon and the hypothalamus.

It seems evident that the frontal portion of the cerebral cortex exerts a modifying and stabilizing influence on the nerve centers in the hypothalamus. If these centers are disconnected by dissection in the laboratory, or through atrophy from improper blood nourishment, the result is violent and uncontrollable rage elicited by slight provocation.

The central nervous system is composed of two parts: the brain, located inside the skull; and the spinal cord, located inside the column of vertebrae. The brain and spinal cord are connected together by nerve tracts passing through the foramen magnum, which is a large hole situated at the base of the skull. The brain is the operating part of the central nervous system containing nearly all of the nerve cells in that system. The spinal cord is composed mainly of nerve tracts going to or away from the brain, being called efferent or afferent tracts respectively. The spinal cord contains billions of nerve tracts grouped in large ascending and descending columns in the spinal cord. The size, shape, and location of these columns have been chronicled accurately and named. However, a detailed knowledge of spinal cord configuration is of no direct value to our understanding of the operation of the neural system. This knowledge is of course of inestimable importance to neurosurgeons and to youngsters preparing for their state board examinations in allopathy (medicine), chiropractic, osteopathy, and naturopathy.

The spinal cord is similar in a way to a telephone cable containing an incomprehensibly large number of fine wires carrying intelligence. The spinal cord is wrapped in several coverings and is free to move within the vertebral canal of the spinal column as that column flexes and bends.

The spinal cord throws thirty-one pairs of spinal nerves in the average human individual. These spinal nerves exit the spinal column through spinal foramina or nerviducts. As the individual bends and flexes in his daily routine, consisting of such things as getting into the family automobile and out again, the spinal nerves must move slightly in the nerviducts. If the spinal nerves do not slip in the nerviduct as the spinal column flexes, the spinal cord and spinal nerves appended may be stretched and perhaps damaged. A freely flexible vertebral column together with properly operating spinal nerviducts is essential. Undesirable stretching of our nerve tracts in the spinal cord will occur if spinal nerves cannot slide freely in nerviducts as our spine is flexed and extended.

The peripheral nervous system is a simple and straightforward system. It consists of nerve tracts going to or from nerve cell bodies in the brain. It connects the regulatory nerve cell sections in the brain with distant tissues by outgoing nerve tracts. Incoming nerve tracts bring sensory messages to nerve cell sections in the brain.

The peripheral nerve system can be divided in several different ways for ease in study. Thus, the peripheral system can be said to be composed of twelve cranial nerves, and about thirty-one pairs of spinal nerves. The cranial nerves pass directly from the brain through various holes in the bottom and sides of the skull. The spinal nerves, implicit as nerve tracts in the spinal cord, exit the spinal column through thirty-one pairs of flexible nerviducts; of course the sacral nerviducts are not flexible later in life. The twelve cranial nerves proceed directly to their destination without any ganglionic relay stations. However, part of nerves leaving by way of the thirty-one pairs of spinal nerviducts require ganglionic relay stations. The sympathetic nerves which exit from the twelve thoracic and upper two or three lumbar nerviducts proceed to a section of the nervous system known as the sympathetic gangliated chain. This chain runs parallel to the spinal column and contains groupings of nerve cells which act as relay points for sympathetic nerve tracts. After the sympathetic nerves (which were known as preganglionic sympathetic nerves before they reached the chain) leave the sympathetic chain, they are referred to as postganglionic sympathetic nerve fibers. There is no special difference between postganglionic nerve fibers and preganglionic nerve fibers since they are an integral part of the same system performing an identical function.

Spinal nerve tracts which leave the spinal cord by way of the spinal nerviducts throw some branches which do not go to the gangliated chain. These nerve tracts proceed directly to their destination in muscles, bones, etc. These nerves are a part of the peripheral nervous system but are separate from the sympathetic nerves which pass through relay points on their way to the viscera.

Peripheral nerve branches which pass to the sympathetic chain are a part of the autonomic nervous system. Those nerves not proceeding to the chain for onward relay are a part of the cerebro spinal system. This is an undesirable name and perhaps confusing because those autonomic nerves which pass through the sympathetic chain are also a part of the cerebro spinal system.

A further division of the neural system brings us to the sympathetic and parasympathetic segments of the autonomic or visceral nervous system. The parasympathetic or craniosacral nervous system leaves the central nervous system by way of the third, seventh, ninth, tenth, and eleventh cranial nerves, and the second, third, and fourth sacral spinal nerves. The sympathetic or thoracolumbar overflow leaves as we have already noted by the thoracic and first two or three lumbar spinal nerves.

It is sufficient for us to know that the brain contains the nerve control centers. The spinal cord and peripheral nerves simply consist of nerve tracts connected to the brain cells at one end, and our body on the other end. Our body cells can be visceral, bony, muscular, glandular, visual, etc.

The brain system (brain, spinal cord, and peripheral nerves), then, is the first system to be laid out in clearly identifiable relief, and in distinct detail in earliest fetal stages. As long as the brain system retains its perfect integrity, so also will all other nonneural tissues of the body remain perfect, distinctly formed, and operationally faithful to original plan. However, should the neural system fail to function perfectly, so also will other associated nonneural tissues of the body lose their distinct shape and functional capability.

With cerebellar perfection we enjoy somatic symmetry, beauty, and grace. With brain impairment we suffer somatic tissue irregularity, discomfort, fatigue, and chronic illness of all sorts, types and classifications. With brain perfection, all nonneural tissues feel distinct and fully animated. With brain trauma, tissues feel indistinct and incompletely animated.

So the sense of this chapter is this: the brain system is the prime material system of our physical body. It takes distinct shape from the very beginning, and controls the development of nonneural tissues into a somatic human body. Later in life, if parts or all of the brain system become impaired, the associated nonneural tissues will degenerate. Thus, if facial nerves are affected, the somatic tissues of the face will lose their distinct shape. The distinct lip line will vanish, the face will sag prematurely, deep lines will form, the face may bloat, become haggard, or cancerous, depending on other companion neural problems, in distant areas of the body. That which holds true for the face also pertains to all nonneural somatic areas such as the liver, kidneys, heart, lungs, legs, arms, hips, or spine itself.

It is demonstrably evident that the human individual in its earliest stages contains primitive tissues which are to subsequently elaborate, forming the tissues and organs of our body.

Moreover, it is palpably discernible that the brain system expands and develops at a much more rapid rate in the beginning than the neighboring nonneural somatic tissue.

All bones which surround the nerves are formed after the brain system has been formed. Thus, the holes in the cranium and spinal cord are not formed first, and the nerves do not later thread their way through the osseous foramen en route to vital organs. Rather, the nerves are laid out first in precise detail and exquisite shape, and the cartilage and bones of the skull and vertebrae are formed later around the brain system.

PART 2

The brain is the central engine of man.

Inanimate engines are vastly less complicated than animated organisms. The simplest inanimate engine is a loop knot in a piece of string. The structure of the knot functions to shorten the string, increase its mass at the juncture of the knot, and provides feedback monitoring of tension with tightening because the string is reflected upon itself. The content of the knot is string. There is an input into the knot and an energy output when the opposite ends of the string containing the knot are manipulated.*

Living creatures are constructed of materials which constitute their content. They receive an input, produce an output. They are provided with a feedback circuitry in the brain, which controls through the monitoring of activity. As is the case with all engines, excessive structural alteration will swing the range of function into a distorted area and adversely modify the content of the device. It can even impair the ability of the structure to receive a normal input or transmit a normal output.

In the more complicated living engines such as man, there are several organic systems all of which are integrated to make the complete person in human form. Here the chances for structural distortion of an interlocking nature are greater than in less complicated devices or life forms. Man is perhaps the most important engine in nature. Yet he is more than an ordinary engine because he has some control over himself.

Pleneurethic's pentifacet with field of parallel lines in five directions stands for a creature of nature or engine of man.

The first facet represents *input* into the pentifacet. Parallel lines are drawn toward the opposite facet which represents the *structural* aspect of any device of nature or man.

*See Fig. 2.

If the structure is proper, fine parallel lines will be reflected to another facet which stands for the *function*.

From there the lines are again reflected to the facet which represents the *content* of any device. If the content is proper an *output* will be achieved.

Lines from the output facet are reflected back to the original facet—this feedback is present in all devices and is necessary for control and monitoring of operation.

The Pleneurethical Star emerges automatically if the pentifacet is proper and all lines have been correctly reflected. Thus the star is not drawn in or constructed, but arises spontaneously as a result of perfection in the device. We as humans will exhibit the Pleneurethical Star only when we have perfected ourselves.

The pentifacet was originally derived by installing a simple loop knot in a strip of paper and then carefully flattening the knot.

The circle around the pentifacet symbolizes Pleneurethic at work in the world.

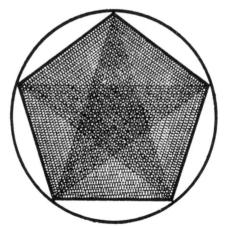

Fig. 2.   THE PENTIFACET

As we all have observed from the operation of mechanical engines, engines can be overloaded. The brain can also be overloaded.

Loading may be imposed upon central neural resources by mentality. It may also be presented to the brain by stimuli which vibrate through the normal sensory receptors. Such loading is normal. It may be light or excessively heavy but it is nevertheless normal and may be avoided if the person wishes to avoid it. Problems can be forgotten. It is possible to move away from loud noises or else plug the ears to shut them out. People dislike mental frustration because it places a temporary load on the brain.

The extra burden that is imposed on the brain by a frustrated mentality can acutely diminish its overall vigor and buoyance and can attenuate the enjoyment of life. If the frustration is prolonged or intensified it may threaten the survival potential of the individual and may even destroy its basis for life.

Abnormal loading may also be forced upon the brain by a disorder in the bioductory system. This type of loading can only be described as chronic. It is reduced when the brain and the body are resting but there can never be any complete escape from it. In time this type of loading causes the brain to deteriorate, or in mechanical terms, to run down.*

Because the loading is chronic it continues to impose itself on the brain even after the brain has begun to deteriorate under its pressure. As it builds up, chronic illness strikes the body and brings in its train premature death.

Such loading is abnormal. It cannot be evaded by the stricken person or the stricken brain. The body's sensory system is not equipped to indicate the source of trouble to the brain because nature neglected to supply the neural system with a method of determining the exact location of trauma along the surface of major tracts of the neural system itself.

Chronic loading on the brain or chronic illness cannot improve automatically by itself. The condition, however, as interpreted by the sufferer will be characterized by cyclic periods of exacerbation and remission with perhaps gently declivitous plateaus in between.

*See Fig. 3.

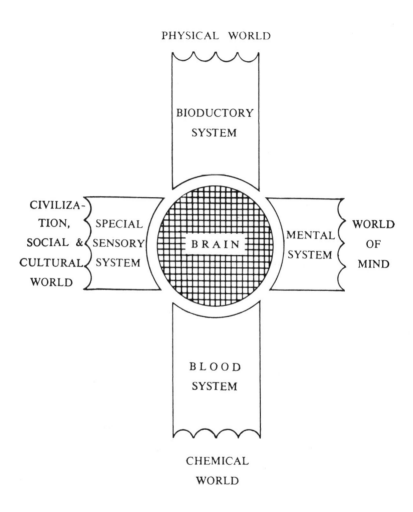

Fig. 3. SYSTEM OF CEREBELLAR COAXIALITIES

Brain with four coaxial relationships: neurophysical, neuromental, neurochemical, and neurosocial. A malstructure anywhere in the system establishes stresses which are transmitted by brain to all other portions of the system.

54

Even if the afflicted person recognizes the fact that his bioductory system is causing undue strain on his brain and body he is unable to correct the cause himself. Because the disorder results from traumatized, malpostured, hypomobile areas of the bioductory system the condition requires external force applied by an intelligent operator to relieve it. It can only be cured through treatment administered in the Pleneurethical manner.

The original prime disorder that produced the chronic illness was induced painfully through physical shock. Therefore, the restoration process must commence with a correctional reordering force which will also be painful.

We hasten to add that any general manipulative force applied haphazardly and indiscriminately to the area of the spinal injury will also produce pain. It will also produce temporary stimulation through irritating the tissues. It will not, however, be corrective in nature unless it precisely reorders the immobilized bioducts.

The concept of the bioductory system and the axial prominence of the brain is the vital factor which separates Pleneurethic from other healing disciplines. In Pleneurethic the bioduct concept takes in much more than the bony regions of the spine. It also concerns itself with the neural system which travels to the muscle and ligamentous tissues of the body.

It should be noted that, as the neural system is restored to order under Pleneurethical care, resulting regeneration will occur more or less simultaneously in exactly the same areas that chronic degeneration occurred. Thus, as the trend of the chronic illness is reversed the old symptoms will reappear in reverse order to their original appearance.

For example, take the case of a young boy who fell and injured his bioductory structure in a manner which was to affect the lower right side of his body. His right hip was directly injured in the fall. As it was knocked out of position, it took the lumbar area of the bioductory system with it. This placed pressure on the spinal cord, brain, and spinal nerves, which built up into progressive trauma as time passed.

Because of the way the hip was pushed out of alignment, the right leg system became half an inch shorter than the left leg.

Pain developed in the left leg and left hip as they adapted themselves to having to take an increased proportion of the body's
weight distribution. The vast anatomical rearrangement which was
made necessary because of the accident caused the boy to suffer
various pains which occurred on and off during childhood. Some
of these pains were simply a result of the mechanical changes
in the leg system. Other pains were due to neural pathology
resulting from bioductory trauma. After he first had the accident,
the boy limped. But the limp disappeared as he learned to compensate for the injury by allowing his spine to curve sideways.
After growing to manhood he developed kidney, prostate, and
bladder difficulties, impotence, rapid wasting of leg muscles, with
partial paralysis and some arthritis in the low back, hips, and
legs.

Pleneurethical treatment begun before the right leg became
totally and irreversibly crippled would have had the following
effect. As the nerves in the lower bioductory region were rejuvenated, and the abnormal loading on the brain diminished, a
lot of regenerative activity in the lower lumbar hip and leg regions
would be observed. First of all, the lower region of the bioductory
system would develop a normal order. Then the right hip would
move forward into its proper position, making the right hip
and leg of equal length to the left. Next, the joints of the
leg would shift slightly and return to a normal position when
walking. Even the feet would assume a new postural alignment. Lastly, the muscles and ligaments would readapt themselves
and strengthen.

All of these changes would be accompanied by strange
new regenerative pains as muscles which previously were not
used began to work. Unaccustomed pains would also develop
in the joints of the foot, leg, and hip as new surfaces were
brought into use as the leg and hip linkage systems shifted
back to normal. These new patterns of pain would actually be
the earlier "growing" pains of youth being reexperienced and
reencountered following the lower spinal bioductory correction.
Last, but not least, gratifying changes would also be noted in the
tissues of the urinary and genital systems and in the pelvic region
in general.

Very often people suffer damage to the bioductory system in the neck and shoulder areas due to faulty obstetrics, athletic field injuries, etc.

Chronic trauma in the bioductory system of the neck and shoulder area often results in degeneration of tissues in the arms and hands, lungs and heart, and can cause arms and shoulders to become unequal. The condition can cause chronic brain changes which are even more frightening in their manifestations throughout the body and mind. Chronic anxiety ensues, with proclivity to heart attack.

In females mammary gland changes, such as lumps and nodules, may sometimes be noticed.

The outward appearance of such bioductory distortion includes: one shoulder shorter and higher than the other; one arm longer than the other; tension in the sterno cleido mastoidieus muscle of the neck. Motor discoordination in walking may also be noticed, along with nightmares and various forms of severe chronic illnesses.

Pain caused through Pleneurethical treatment is useful and unavoidable, even though it may be at first unwelcomed by the patient. This is particularly so if the patient does not understand its cause and beneficial implications. But the pain is a welcome sign of recovery from the previous degenerative process. Degenerated tissues, which at the beginning of Pleneurethical care were painless, may become exquisitely painful as paralysis and immobility begin to lift and as neurological communication is restored to the stricken region. The patient must understand the reason for such occurrences.

Degenerative pain is a natural result of structural and functional degeneration. Regenerative pain is also a natural process.

This action can be illustrated by taking a fresh prune and subjecting it to a hot and dry desiccating current of air on a drying stand. The skin of the prune puckers as the water is slowly drawn from the fruit. The desiccating atrophy of the prune under such conditions is inescapable, for it is based on the physics of the transfer of fluids from a dense to a less dense substance across a suitable intermediating membrane. When the atrophied, puckered, withered prune is placed in a glass of water a reverse process begins.

Water is drawn across the membranous skin of the prune to the less concentrated state within the prune. The prune slowly absorbs moisture and once again nearly approximates its prior fresh state. This expanding process would be painful if the prune possessed a neural system and cerebellar interpretive center. The transformation is not perfect because the prune is no longer living, having been plucked from the living tree. But, the process through which the atrophied prune takes water from the glass of water surrounding it is inescapable, predictable, and vigorous, for it is based on the mechanics of absolute laws.

The same type of thing happens to somatic flesh in the arms or legs or to a specific area of somatic tissue such as a gland or heart wall that has atrophied chronically and is subsequently restored to normal by Pleneuretical methods. Such atrophy may be caused by chronic loss of neural sufficiency by having been detached in some manner or another from the neural tree.

Inexorable and *brutal* are the terms that best explain the determined degeneration of tissues once their source of neural energy has been chronically curtailed or injuriously tampered with.

As sufficient neural energy is resupplied to the stricken part, *inexorable, inescapable, predictable,* and *brutal* are also the best terms to describe the ruthless manner through which the atrophied flesh is rejuvenated.

As the process of rejuvenation progresses the area becomes swollen (compared to its former emaciated state) and the regenerating tissues are often exquisitely sensitive as they split apart, expand, and dilate as the incoming rush of blood forces them to return to their former voluptuous state. The Pleneurethic regenerative process can be absolutely painful, sometimes pleasurably so, as old areas of emaciated degeneration resume their proper function and receive the buoyant force of life through the violent influx of vital fluids.

Functional regenerative pain may often be spectacular, intense, unexpected, and often difficult to explain.

Bioductory damage can cause brain damage and lead to mental as well as physical problems, which affect the individual's behavior. These mental problems can show early signs of senility. Surprisingly, once the physical problem which led to the undermining of mental stability is corrected, the mental problem adjusts itself and appears to clear itself automatically.

Chronic damage to an area of the bioductory system causes chronic damage to the correlative portion of the neural system, and this pathological process is termed *bioductosis* and *neuralosis* respectively.

Pleneurethical discussions with actual chronically ill patients reveal a faithful continuity of symptoms often stemming from early childhood. In some cases the intense earaches of infancy progressively graduate into numbness of the external ear, ringing of the inner ear, and headaches later in life. The afflicted person may feel so tormented that he may even wish to remove his offending ear like the painter Van Gogh, who cut off his ear after voluntarily committing himself to institutions for the insane on several occasions.

In other cases, the painful low back and hip experienced in early chilhood can become growing pains in adolescence, and finally arthritic and paralytic later in life. Once a neuralotic syndrome is established it never really relents, but continues to worsen as it proceeds through a predictable and orderly course of tissue degeneration and intellectual functional impairment.

The only known remedy for conditions caused by this syndrome is the restoration of brain sufficiency through bioductory restructuring, following Pleneurethical procedures. A cure definitely does not lie in any one of the large range of variations on the talking- or thinking-type approach to healing which is usually adopted toward the chronically ill. These approaches can cause more harm to the person because they sometimes reinforce the guilt syndrome that often accompanies chronic illness. This is particularly so in cases where the psychotherapist overemphasizes matters of sex.

It is abhorrent, presumptuous, and bordering on the depraved for a psychotherapist to ask female patients who are suffering from the real and crushing impact of chronic illness, how it feels to engage in coitus and questions relating to undignified sexuality.

At best such discussions can only shock or temporarily stimulate a sick person.

Most people are not obsessed with sex, as some analysts demonstrate themselves to be. There is an entire universe of ideas and notions which inhabit the mentality of people, of which sex may play but a small part. This is especially true when people suffer desperate degrees of chronic illness.

Pleneurethical diagnosis and restructuring of bioductory disorders and intellectual malstructures proceed equally well with men and women, with children and old people, with dull and intelligent people, with the poor and with the rich, without such discussions. This shows it is unnecessary to discuss intimate details of oral, anal, genital, or phallic stages in order to produce a cure. Not only are such discussions unnecessary but they are undesirable because they waste time and serve no useful purpose in the majority of cases. Some acute mental afflictions have their basis in a structural degeneration of the mentality, and are not in any way due to physical impairment of the neural system. They are problems that are caused through the undermining of the patient's ethical nature.

For example, the Pleneurethical interpretation of the term *psychosis* may be demonstrated by a young man, with fixed ideas about nonviolence, who is forced to invade another nation and slaughter its inhabitants. Before this event the mentality of the youth was structured with notions of nonviolence and brotherly love. However, in the war situation he is ordered to slaughter his human opponent. If he does not kill he will in turn be killed for disobeying military authority. To be able to carry out these orders he has to change the attitude of his mind so that it accepts that what was once good has become bad. What was monstrously bad and evil has become good and necessary for his survival. In the process the basic structure of his mentality is demolished. His personality is ripped apart between his intellectual guidelines and his physical actions.

A psychosis is likely to develop because the youth cannot

satisfactorily restructure his intellectual mentality to cope with the realities of his situation. As a result the youth could develop a psychotic condition in which his behavior is acutely modified as are some of his somatic functions. He may experience physical side effects which include acute indigestion, a loss of appetite, sleeplessness, and a feeling of debility and uneasiness.

The treatment for such a problem is verbal. It is in the realm of ideas, notions, and the squaring of the patient's aspirations with reality.

The great and heartbreaking tragedy of present-day psychotherapy is that it makes no meaningful discrimination between such things as: acute anxiety and simple immature withdrawal due to some social reverse; and chronic withdrawal, apathy, and total defeat from a grinding neuralosis and bioductory disorder which shatters brain competence.

Most practicing psychotherapists lack the training and insight required to separate acute anxiety from chronic anxiety. In the eyes of most psychotherapists the acute anxiety which comes from concern over job failure due to a poor education appears no different from free-floating apprehension, guilt, and job failure which stems from severe neural insufficiency caused by a bioductory disorder.

Therefore, some psychotherapists who enjoy relative success in treating cases of simple social maladjustment cannot understand why the same treatment fails utterly in the treatment of other apparently similar cases of maladjustment. Because of their training they are unable to appreciate that these cases are actually different because they arise from a chronic physical cause and not purely from an acute mental disturbance.

Psychotherapy can bring temporary stimulation to a person suffering from chronic mental and physical illness but it cannot bring about a permanent restoration of the patient's mental faculties. Pleneurethic can do this if the corrective process is begun before the brain cells themselves are irreversibly damaged by fever and delirium.

Many chronically ill patients do not respond well to psychiatric treatment. Often, when the psychological approach eventually proves fruitless, sufferers are kept dangling by being told that their illnesses are spurious, specious, and imaginary. They may be told that their mental processes are totally and hopelessly deranged but that further psychological processing may succeed in unlocking the door to instantaneous physical health. After years of costly analytical processing they may be dropped from processing groups as being hopeless nonresponders. They can also be viciously indicted as being people who prefer to be ill because they have no real wish to be well. In this way, the chronic illness sufferer is often denounced by the same psychotherapist who accepted his case in the first place on the basis of a mind-over-matter cure.

To cope with some of the severe mental derangements which can grow out of chronic illness, horrible, gross, and crude practices have developed. These include: the draining away of spinal fluid; shock, either chemically or electrically induced, which produces bone-shattering and nerve-ending convulsions; and brain-scrambling operations through hideous prefrontal lobotomies.

PART 3

The psyche (mind) receives as much attention in Pleneurethic as does the body, because both affect cerebellar microstructure and influence resistance to disease. Restructuring the body's bioductory system is perhaps more dramatic in its accomplishment than restructuring the psyche, but mental restructuring may indeed be most significant in some cases.

Psychic structure, and its bilateral relationship with the brain, is exceptionally important in determining potential for health and mental attainment. Much of the basis for Pleneurethic's astonishing success is derived from its emphasis upon development and refinement of the individual's *psychic structure* through a special restructuring process. Both the process and the phrase, *psychic structure,* are unique to Pleneurethic. The study and practice of psychic restructuring takes the student into the realm of the spiritual as well as the temporal. Now, while in the realm of the temporal, we must not fail to consider the role of earthy bacteria in the health-versus-disease process.

Pleneurethic postulates that microorganisms, by themselves, are never the first cause of chronic disease. Pathogenic bacteria may be collaterally present in specific cases of chronic illness, but they cannot logically be accused of precipitating the entire chronic condition. Thus, *Staphylococcus aureus* may be present at the site of an acute knife wound, but these bacteria were not the cause of the knife wound. Similarly, *Streptococcus pyogenes* may be found in the tissues of a chronic sore throat, but they were not the cause of the sore throat. This disease comes from cervical bioductory disorder and its depressing and pathological effect on central neurological tissues.

Treponema pallidum may be present in cases of rash, debility, and deterioration of the central neural system. But this type of bacteria does not cause the chronic set of symptoms popularly subsumed under the rubric of syphilis. Rather, an extensive structural disorder of the central bioductory and neurological system causes the symptoms of syphilis, including the somatic condition which allows the proliferation of a form of bacteria found in the diseased body. In such cases, central bioductory trauma is destroying the brain and spinal cord through a process of depleneurization. This in turn causes chronic mental and physical symptoms, and permits incubation of bacteria peculiar to the medical disease termed syphilis. This is not to say that an acute case of syphilis cannot be contracted from exposure to a person with a chronic condition. But the acute case will be just that, and will never manifest the potential for total deterioration exhibited by a chronic case. Bacteria, then, may complicate an area of chronic disaster once it has occurred, but they do not cause it in the first place. Therefore, sanitation and medication may forestall complications, but further sanitation and medication is not in itself curative of chronic illness.

A well-structured body and psyche maintain adequate levels of neural energy in the brain. Neurological capability may diminish as geriatric age increases, but it does so in an orderly and non-pathological and natural manner. Pathogenic bacteria are unable to become a chronic problem, even in old age, if neurological resources are normal.

4

BRAIN-MIND RELATIONSHIP

PART 1

In one way or another, the brain acts and reacts to all internal and external events which touch the body or reach the mind. By placing the brain at the axis of my philosophy, I have opened a new area of reality and made it easier to study and understand the interrelations between many superficially differentiated fields including, for example, physiology, anthropology, sociology, religion, and mysticism.

The person with an unblemished central neural system will be basically happy, but the person whose central neural system is under heavy bioductory assault will be basically unhappy and thoroughly depressed, with a tendency to bad dreams and inaccurate perceptions of reality, no matter how fortunate his other circumstances.

The object of Pleneurethic is environmental management to produce optimum brain capability in the individual and to extend the benefits of this to embrace the community, the nation, and ultimately the world.

Optimum brain performance demands good ethic and constructive intellect. The individual reflecting this represents the minimum basic unit on which to build our hopes for the survival and progress of our present civilization. No matter how great a person's neurological gift, it will amount to nothing unless it is effectively managed. Many people fritter away neurological resources when they are young and their energy seems inexhaustible. In middle age, they rationalize their failure to achieve their goals in life by blaming the economic system, the upper class, another seemingly more privileged race, or other convenient scapegoat such as male chauvinist pigs.

Neurological resources can also be frittered away, and to discover how it is interesting to study the brain-mind bilateral relationship from the perspective of dreams, which play an invaluable role in ridding the brain of tension.

Tension accumulates in brain tissue where it is retained until dissipated or removed. The more tension is accumulated the more the brain is occupied in dealing with it and the less capacity it has for coping with any new demands that are made on it. Cerebellar tension may come from unresolved intellectual problems; from mechanical bioductory trauma acting on the central neural system's nerve tracts at the base of the brain or in the spinal cord and its peripheral extensions; from sensory receptors at the sensitive endings of the various nerve tracts; from poisons, either consumed or absorbed from outside the body; or from toxins generated from within the body by the chronic illness process.

When one goes to bed, the brain and mind move progressively from a state of semisleep where daydreams can occur to complete and actual dreams. Daydreams and "night" dreams are mental reflections of a relaxing brain relieving itself of stress accumulated during the day. When bioductosis destroys the structural and mechanical integrity of the bioductory system in whole or in part, the central neurological system does not shed its level of stress as it should. In fact, the bioductosis causes accumulation of additional, heavier than normal, levels of chronic cerebellar stress or neuralosis.

This is why nightmares occur. The brain is trying to relax itself but it cannot because it is being chronically irritated by confused signals from the main nerve tracts in the body. The brain's effort is reflected into the mind to cause a vague but frightening basis for nightmare during sleep and chronic anxiety while awake.

The normal dream is based on acute cerebellar tension caused by episodes involving intellectual conflict. By contrast, nightmares are produced by chronic neurological trauma and tension resulting from a chronic mechanical and physical impact on the bioductory system which is registered on a nonverbal level in the brain.

Dream themes are elicited by and tend to follow the pattern of social and intellectual events of the preceding days. Nightmares reflect accidents which destroyed bioductory structural symmetry, which may have occurred decades earlier, sometimes as long ago as malobstetrics at birth. Nightmare themes are bizarre and hectic because the mind finds it difficult to impute a suitable verbal or social interpretation to violent and mechanically induced brain turbulence caused by chronic trauma received on a subverbal level.

There is a close relationship between hysteria and dreams, but not of the sort most professional and lay people have been led to believe.

Freud, and the schools of psychology indebted to him, believed that dreams were entirely of a psychological genesis resulting from hostile desire, repressed wish, and other mechanisms resident in the mind. Conventional psychologists, of whatever school, endeavor to pierce the mystery of dreams by free association and other purely verbal-mental techniques.

Approaching the analysis of dreams in this way, conventional psychologists have consistently missed a vitally significant point. They have been focusing their attention on the content of the dream. In other words, they have been concentrating on its trivial surface aspects. Thus, they are completely engrossed in interpreting such things as receptacles, valleys, and crevices as vaginas, and elongated objects such as pointers, projections, and weapons spurting deadly material, as symbolic penises.

In Pleneurethic this type of analysis is considered unreliable as an approach to curing chronic illness. The idea in curing any disease is to remove the cause, not to use the symptoms as a vehicle for demonstrating intellectual virtuosity before the eyes of the "doctor's" dying patients.

The Pleneurethical approach in healing is to remove all sources contributing to an accumulation of unconstructive stress in the central neurological tissues. Since the brain provides the power for thought and range of mind together with coordination of somatic organic activity, it is essential that it retains optimum neurological capability by remaining free from unconstructive tension.

The portion of the brain associated with conscious thought becomes awake and operative when sufficient rest has been secured and this is the time to get out of bed and to begin to perform the tasks of the day. But, in upper bioductory trauma (suboccipital, cervical, and upper thoracic bioductosis), the brain is chronically upset and unable to function properly. The degree of the upset depends on the severity of the ailment and the length of time it has had to deteriorate. This has the effect of destroying the usefulness of the normal test of the proper time to get up in the morning.

Indeed, a turbulent state of the brain may deny the body proper sleep and substitute a hellish nocturnal state of affairs. When this happens, nightmarish, fitful, very light sleep occurs and the conscious mind may continue to function on and off during the entire night. To describe this state, a new term was introduced into Pleneurethical terminology. The new term is *pleneurity*. It means a condition of complete neurological normalcy in the brain and the remainder of the central and peripheral neural system. When the brain is partially depleted and its actions become abnormal as a result of cerebellar tension, it is depleneurized. When the cause of all the improper and unconstructive tension has been removed, the brain is repleneurized and able to function normally.

If the brain were depleneurized by a heavy acute effort, which could be described in words complete with heavy mental tension and conflict, the dream sequence of the following night would, quite probably, parallel the tension-producing event.

Supposing an individual during the course of the day needed to keep a number of very important appointments in different parts of the city and to keep them he had to dash from one place to another by taxi. The difficulty in getting taxis when he wanted them, coupled with a series of brain-tensing encounters during the interviews, might be followed by dream sequences reflecting the day's activities, as the brain repleneurized itself from acute tension developed during the day.

If the same person was suffering from increasingly chronic

brain tension brought about by deteriorating bioductory trauma, the events of the day could bring him hell in the night. For him the stage is set for nightmare and a host of other ailments which complete the chronic depleneurization syndrome.

The sleeping brain might produce a pattern of instability which could be interpreted by the mind as a terrifying wild taxi ride interspersed with numerous tension-producing and fear-inducing episodes as the mind retreats in time and recalls other traumatic experiences which could have been easily verbalized when they occurred. The events of the day had been super-imposed on persistent brain turbulence of nonintellectual, sub-verbal, chronic bioductory origin. This superimposition makes it possible to explain a number of perplexing things. Chief among them is how psychiatry or prayer can often improve a seriously ill patient to a certain point, but cannot prevent the patient's death.

The explanation is simple if we consider that cerebellar tension builds up cumulatively like the layers of an onion.

Let us examine how a seriously ill patient, suffering from heavy neurological stress springing from several different sources, responds to treatment.

If his diet is corrected and he is gotten off tobacco and alcohol and given some tonic or stimulant, his condition will show some improvement. He may even feel that he is cured and may even be convinced that he is, especially if he is assured that there is now nothing wrong with him. But a few months later the anxious feeling of unwellness returns and he knows that there is something wrong with him. He does not know precisely what it is so he goes to see a psychiatrist or a clergyman. After he puts his faith into the suggestive verbal therapy they have to offer his tension load becomes further lightened and he once again feels cured, this time, properly. But the feeling of unwellness returns and with it anxiety. In time the patient knows that a hard core of tension exists in his being and it is punishing him to death. This last hard core is central physioneurological stress from neuralosis—the final layer of the onion of tension.

It is caused by a bioductory disorder. If it is peeled off through Pleneurethical restructuring processes the patient will be well and whole again, as long as fever and delirium have not destroyed parts of the brain before Pleneurethical treatment was begun.

Only a person with Pleneurethical training can tell whether physioneurological tension exists in the central brain system and the extent of it. He is also in a position to know whether the mental condition should be cured physically through mechanical correction of bioductory torsion or through verbal methods aimed at straightening out a malstructured intellect.

According to Pleneurethical philosophy, anxiety, acute or chronic, is nature's way of advising an individual that something is dangerously wrong. When the welfare of the person is openly menaced, acute anxiety will persist until the dangerous situation has abated or is understood. When a satisfactory course of action has been adopted and the threat to the person has subsided, the acute anxiety will dissipate with a feeling of relief. Anxiety is an unpleasant sensation and will persistently advise the individual of the existence of a potentially harmful situation until corrective action has been taken. Because of this it has some relationship to pain. Both indicate that something is endangering the person's security and chances of survival. Both sensations are perfectly normal.

Before Pleneurethic, chronic anxiety was unfortunately thought to be baseless and abnormal. It was mistakenly thought to exist for no reason other than a bizarre and perverse distortion of the imagination in the mind of a malingering and unresponsive pseudo-sufferer.

The treatment for chronic anxiety was, then, to persuade the patient to "straighten up" his thinking. This treatment was ineffective because it was directed not at the prime cause of the condition but at the symptoms.

There is a multitude of chronic mental anxiety cases which appear to non-Pleneurethically-oriented people to have arisen for no good reason. The history is the same in each case. The person was normal or nearly so during childhood. Then gradually the chronic symptoms appeared. Slowly at first, so that only the sufferer was aware of them and then often only vaguely so, but later becoming so prominent that they could not be hidden from even casual acquaintances.

Pleneurethic can only restore people to their normal state. If normalcy is idiocy, Pleneurethic is helpless. It cannot create capability where it did not already exist.

Through Pleneurethic we know that the type of chronic anxiety previously referred to as abnormal is actually very normal because it springs from a direct and very real cause. This is a pathologically damaged major nerve tract which adversely affects parent cell bodies in the brain in diverse physiological ways.

Chronic anxiety seldom occurs alone, and is usually accompanied by a family of related negative emotions which form a syndrome. There is a great variety of these lesser emotions and they may be experienced in greater or lesser degrees depending on the location and extent of the bioductory trauma and the habits of the individual.

The chronically anxious person is emotionally disturbed by relatively trivial events, especially in cases of severe cervical and upper thoracic bioductory disorder. In the early stages it is difficult to distinguish the emotional disturbance from normal merriment or a zest for living. Children may become hyperactive and difficult to manage in the classroom. However, as it approaches the maniacal, it becomes uncontrollable.

The other extreme of excitement is depression and apathy, and here again it is difficult to discriminate between a normal gloomy period following an actual disappointment and the beginning of chronic moody depression.

Hostility and anger also become companion symptoms of some chronic anxiety patients. We find these patients indulging in anger, hostility, and aggressive acts out of all proportion to the external event which triggered the emotional outburst of the moment.

Hypersensitivity occurs uniformly in varying degrees of severity in all chronic anxiety cases. In almost all cases of chronic anxiety and hypersensitivity we find the individual to be suffering from constant and unabated brain assault brought about by improperly functioning sections of the bioductory system. This condition maintains a persistent physical trauma on the central neural system, causing an irritable and hyperstimulated condition of tension in the brain of the sufferer and even reduces blood supply to the brain or spinal cord on some occasion.

Thus, as the condition worsens, genuine (not imaginary) feelings of apprehension, worry, and fear appear.

The time required for the transition from the first signs of worry and fear into the final flight of deep apprehension and abject terror may require months, years, or decades, depending on the severity of the bioductory trauma and other factors too numerous to mention. However, in some cases, only a few days are required for the ailment to proceed to a violent crisis followed by immediate death or a prolonged period of varying degrees of living death.

Structural distortion of the bioductory system may not only bring concomitant neurological distortion and loss of mental confidence, it may also evoke a loss of self-respect and self-esteem. The mechanism is very simple. As the level of personal capability declines, the sufferer may grow to detest himself for his incompetence in dealing with things which he had previously undertaken as routine. As a result he feels his business associates no longer treat him as an equal, but rather as one who has proved incapable of running the race. His family in their misunderstanding bestow pity and perhaps contempt as they witness the slow degeneration of their previous hero, provider, and champion. Nothing is left except to meet the inevitable, which is sometimes hastened by efforts at self-destruction.

Such a person may become suspicious of staunch friends or loyal family members. The most heartbreaking aspect of the whole affair is that the more suspicious the sufferer and the more intense his floundering efforts to discover the true source of his ailment, the more he is laughed at and ridiculed as being demented by regular medical professionals. The person knows he is not demented, but how can he explain his condition when no sympathetic ears are trained to understand and treat the basic anatomical cause of his very real neurological disorder.

Another bothersome thing in the psychological ball of anxious twine is excessive mind action. This invariably accompanies chronic anxiety until, toward the end, an exhausted brain is unable to function and registers nothing but apathy or coma, because the brain, in part or in whole, is at the very threshold of collapse and death.

Discussion of the chronic anxiety syndrome cannot be complete until the emotion of insecurity is mentioned. It is one of the most persistent members of the syndrome and prevails in the mind of the afflicted despite his every effort to eliminate it. Long after all problems of outside life have been solved, the feeling of insecurity persists, no matter how often the sufferer tells himself that all is well.

The basic cause of chronic anxiety may be reinforced by other factors.

First, as peripherally associated somatic tissues degenerate in structure and function from their lack of cerebellar communication, they liberate toxins. All of these toxins are not immediately neutralized or eliminated from the body. As the toxin level in the blood rises, the brain becomes increasingly saturated with it. This will contribute to the intensifying of the existing deleterious neural condition as the heavy biomechanical irritation of the brain cells from bioductory strain is biochemically reinforced by the caustic action of poisons from a deteriorating soma (body) on brain tissues.

A second manner in which the reinforcement of chronic neurological pathology is conveyed to the brain is through interferences with Suri's Tract, which regulates the supply of blood to the brain. Bioductory problems can affect Suri's Tract and by so doing will impair and reduce cerebral blood circulation, adding to the already direct pathological abuse to the brain stem and spinal cord caused through the bioductory disorder. As the supply of blood to the brain is reduced its ability to function properly declines. Anxiety, desperation, apprehension, and all of the remaining members of the chronic anxiety syndrome eventually emerge to reinforce the original condition. Accidental damage to the neck and shoulder areas has the potential to cause harm to Suri's Tract.

There is another facet to this problem of chronic anxiety and the usual mental and physical problems accompanying it.

The brain is an organ whose neurological stamina and energy capacity is not unlimited. It is, after all, only a biological tissue and as such is able to do only so much work in a 24-hour day without suffering varying degrees of exhaustion and eventual structural impairment.

Most chronic anxiety sufferers experience rapid relief under Pleneurethical care.

When Pleneurethical treatment is applied to chronic mental disorders I do not ordinarily waste time or the patient's energy in psychically or verbally oriented therapy. Rather, I seek to improve brain performance and elevate the brain's capability by mechanically correcting the physical cause of the brain debility. This is done by locating the region of the bioductory system that is chronically traumatizing the central neural system. Such malstructures in the bioductory system have usually been caused by severe accidents.

The actual correction of bioductory system derangements biomechanically requires a very precise knowledge of the human anatomy and operating expertise by the operator. It is beyond the scope of this book to outline in detail the exact technique in any particular case because every case is different in the nature and degree of bioductory system distortion and deterioration.

Relief comes in two stages. The first stage results from the patient's ability to understand the true source of the malady. As a result they are able to superficially relax because they know that they are not suspected of being mentally deranged, and also because they have been offered a plausible and acceptable solution to their problems. However, this relief is not basic to Pleneurethical treatment and I do not encourage it in my therapeutic treatment program.

The second stage usually makes its appearance within a few days or weeks after Pleneurethical management is commenced. As the intolerable burden of major neurological disorder is removed, the cause of chronic anxiety is rapidly cancelled. An unbelievable feeling of well-being is once again in the grasp of the person as his head feels clearer and lighter and his face appears fresher.

Pleneurethical treatment arrests the cause of chronic illness and reverses its course. The patient then returns to a condition of normalcy for his age. The external symptoms of the illness disappear, to be replaced by normal skin tone. The development of muscles, including those under the skin in the face, in the gastrointestinal tract, and in and around the heart, returns to normal. So does the production of cells in the marrow of the bones. Mental outlook is also improved because it no longer has to try to cope with the terrible drag imposed on it by a deteriorating brain.

The two terms *unconscious* and *subconscious* are widely used in psychotherapy and much dogma is based on their meaning and significance.

Psychotherapists' research indicates that the unconscious mind is the seat of the Id, Ego, and Super Ego. Thus, they suppose it to be the storehouse for sexual energy and the central core of personality drives and desires. To them the unconscious mind also represents all of the mental accumulation acquired through conscious life. And, finally, they regard it as a monitor and guide to action, acquired from experience of childhood plus mother relationships.

Thus, present-day psychotherapeutic meaning of "the unconscious" is so broad that the various authorities have stripped the term of any real meaning, and as a result it is of no real use in diagnostic discussion.

The term *subconscious mind* appears to mean all things referred to by the term *unconscious,* but without specific reference to Id, Ego, and Super Ego. Psychotherapeutic circles disagree on how the word should be used.

The Pleneurethical meaning of "unconscious" is much simpler than that of the psychotherapists. In Pleneurethic, the term is used to refer to a body of thought, memory of past episodes, and ideas which cannot be recalled at any particular time simply by the wish to recall. To the Pleneurethicist, the unconscious mind contains data that once was conscious, but was permitted to sink into the unconscious depths of the mind for storage. The conscious and the unconscious mind are the same mind, but with vertical stratification of memory based on ease of recall. The material on top is of recent acquisition, is easily recalled, and is relatively conscious. Older data which is seldom used is permitted to slide into the bottom strata of the mind where recall is still possible but more difficult because of the psychological distance of the descent.

The mind assigns meaning to brain activity and the process of learning to assign meaning to brain performance is arduous. Indeed, even a lifetime is insufficient for the mind to learn to correctly interpret all of the brain's various signals. Mistakes are often made by the mind in conjuring up a meaning to correspond with brain activity. If brain activity is chronically destabilized because of cerebellar trauma, a normal grasp of reality may never be achieved.

Because of the universal biological position occupied by the brain, it reflects a wide variety of conditions. It is easy for the mind to be misled and to believe that a certain condition is responsible for brain activity when actually another and entirely different condition is responsible. Very often several separate conditions are impacting upon the brain concurrently. If any of the conditions are injuriously bombarding the brain, the mind must discover the cause of the bombardment and abate it. Since the source of some conditions is masked, the mind may impute an erroneous evaluation and aim heroic measures at abatement of the wrong source of trouble.

Pleneurethic discriminates clearly between imagination and material things. Although there is no argument that imagination is a product of our material body and our worldly consciousness in a physical world, imagination in itself is not completely material. If it were, we could replenish our strength upon the imagination of a sumptuous dinner followed by a restful imaginary sleep.

Imagination may lead to a desire for accomplishment, but imagination alone and in itself has no power to directly translate itself into the manipulation of the physics of our material world without the intermediate use of nerves on muscle-moving body levers to meaningfully grasp pick, shovel, or pen. If mind could bypass the brain to work its will in somatic muscles there would be no paralysis.

Also, in Pleneurethic imagination is most emphatically a thing of the temporal world and is not a thing of another foreign, higher, or better world.

Imagination in itself moves no real God and heals no illness other than imaginary illness.

The mind does not tire. It is the brain that becomes exhausted.

It is more correct to say "brain breakdown" than "mental breakdown" or "nervous breakdown." When the brain breaks down the person's behavior becomes even more unpredictable and the attendant sickness reflected in the mind is inevitably accompanied by various chronic illness symptoms in the body.

Our neural system, in part, seems to be a device structured to receive data from outside its confines as conveyed by its peripheral sensors and to transmit this information to a central storage facility. From this facility information may be retrieved by one part of the mind and transmitted to a functioning brain capable of receiving meaningful commands. These commands are sent by means of motor nerves to achieve a desired result in the body and from there to manipulate the external environment.

Brain functioning is work which requires metabolic energy. Many units of neural effort in the brain are required to operate the consciousness of mortal minds.

PART 2

For the purpose of analysis it is possible to divide the psyche into three regions of awareness. These regions are the infraconsciousness (or infrallect), the intellectual consciousness (or intellect), and the supraconsciousness or ultraconsciousness (ultrallect).

Each region of mind is related to an area of the brain. This is in accordance with Pleneurethical postulate.

The infraconsciousness operates mostly below the threshold of ordinary intellectual consciousness and is associated with that part of the brain's activity which presides over the operation of the organs of the body and its blood circulation. The infraconsciousness knows that survival is real and earnest. It is unilaterally intent on survival. It offers no quarter. It is predatory and its roots are deep in the organic earth of the physical body.

By contrast, the ultraconsciousness is all things that the infraconsciousness is not. It is connected with the ethical spirit of our most lofty nature and takes figurative residence with the stars. The ultraconsciousness illuminates our psyche with thoughts of charity, steadfast pure love, and devotion to the service of mankind. Almost everyone can experience some degree of awareness of the ultraconsciousness during the quiet and peaceful periods of inner calm. The ultraconsciousness is also associated with an area of the brain.

In the middle portion of the awareness expanse there is a large mental domain to which I have given the name intellectual consciousness. The intellectual consciousness is associated with the cerebral cortex of the brain and is more or less aware of the existence of the marginal fringes of both the infraconsciousness and the ultraconsciousness. It is also aware of events occurring outside the body which have been reported to it by special sensory organs, and of what it has been taught through formal instruction or by trial and error.

The intellectual consciousness must recognize, coordinate, formulate, and execute plans to carry out its own estimate of whatever situation it finds itself in. At the same time it must entertain the influence of the infraconsciousness and ultra-consciousness as well. The total task of the intellectual consciousness is indeed one of formidable proportions. Perhaps one of its most exciting and complex duties is that of determining a life-work which will be acceptable to at least a part of educated society, which will be economically profitable, and which will bring lifelong satisfaction to the person.

Only the intellect functions in terms of words or concrete pictures. The ultrallect and infrallect deal in sensations and urges. Since the ultrallect does not communicate to one's intellect in trenchant terms of clear prose, the intellect must devise tests to determine the truth and validity of ultrallectual communications.

The difficulty, then, is to determine which of these two regions are are work or whether the function of the intellect is being interfered with by some other aberration of a spurious origin.

The following set of rules can be brought into play to distinguish between them.

The first rule is that the ultrallect never commands. Second, the ultrallect defers to the intellect for a final decision, because the intellect is responsible for the survival of the total individual organism and its successful relationship with the external physical environment. Third, the message of the ultrallect is that of equity, charity of judgment, compassion, and all other ethical virtues. Fourth, communications from the ultrallect are not in terms of specific words or phrases, but rather in terms of a strong desire to subordinate oneself to what may be objectively phrased as grace and honor.

PART 3

In Pleneurethic, I postulate that there is no such thing as an unconscious aspect of mind. Things we see, hear, taste, smell, or learn are never of an unconscious nature. By the very act of knowing with our mind that our brain is transmitting a sensation to the mind, the sensation automatically becomes a conscious perception even though we do not attach a mental meaning to it. The brain may be thought of as being unconscious. The mind, never.

Mentality in Pleneurethic is a product of the interactivity of the brain and the mind. The mind has to evaluate and assign meaning to brain reports concerning the internal and external world. As it establishes a pattern of evaluation for neurological activity, it becomes increasingly structured. Mentality, then, is the part of the mind structured by life experience, but it is more than just pure mind. Pure mind is of little use to anyone until enough of it has been patterned into a responsible and responsive mentality.

Pleneurethic postulates the desirability, necessity, and ability of the individual to influence through mind control the rate of function of the intellect and its basic structure as well.

A major step toward achievement of our ultimate goal is to learn to put the conscious mind and the area of brain inter-relating with it at rest whenever we wish. Once we have mastered the brain and intellect so as to control the rate of their function, we are blessed with a powerful force which may be used to our own advantage and to the constructive benefit of mankind in general. This can be achieved through simple exercises.

Our first exercise begins in some quiet place where there will be no interruptions.

What we will attempt to do is to order the conscious mind and the portion of the brain associated with it to cease to function. It is to lie dormant, motionless, without fluctuation, void of thought. Gradually, with persistence, the mind will remain free of thought for perhaps a few seconds. When this happens one will be well on the way to the point where one can go for a minute or two without finding a single thought flickering across the screen of your intellectual consciousness. The degree of success and length of time taken to achieve it varies vastly among individuals, but if the practice is carried out daily some success will be achieved.

We must next learn to focus the strength of our conscious mentality on but one subject and hold this focus unwaveringly for a definite period. First, we should select some common object such as a small stone, a cloud, a blade of grass, or a flower. If another thought endeavors to invade or replace the pre-meditated subject, we must dismiss it summarily, callously, and decisively. Later, we can expand our comprehension of the subject. We can note its size, shape, color, and everything else of interest about it. We note especially its structure, because truth in Pleneurethic is based upon structural configuration, both macro and micro.

Eventually we can move from concrete objects to the structure of abstract ideas, embodied in such words as *democracy, conservative,* or *god.*

If the student can master these drills he will be well on the way to the development of a Pleneurethical mind, functionally speaking. When he is able to project his entire being into a line of thought for long periods he is able to influence the rate of function of the intellect and its basic structure as well.

How can quality of mind be developed? The answer is not so precise as for the process of developing mental control. But there are several simple drills which will help to elevate the mind's ethical consciousness.

One drill consists of pressing the full power of our intellect, after it has been fashioned for such use by preceding drills, upon such subjects as love, honor, duty, service, and good, as well as allied terms and their opposites.

Another drill to develop quality of ethical mind is to place the mind in a free and open state to receive ennobling motivations from its own ultrallect, its only true source of direct contact with eternal wisdom. Yet another drill to achieve quality of mind is to cross-check various beliefs for validity and fidelity in predicting results.

Quality of mind comes only from deep ethic and does not consist of a surface show of good manners or polished and sophisticated politeness. These are often simply specious facades erected as covers for capricious license and lack of ethical character. Indeed, the reach of high-quality mind is nearly immeasurable by any popular standard. Many people seem peculiarly unable to accurately determine or detect true quality of mind in others.

Some medical practitioners now advocate that a sufferer can cure his own chronic illness by a mental wish to be well. Pleneurethic disagrees with such theories and the therapy that goes with them.

In the chronic illness process the mind does not possess the power to communicate with malpostured sectors of the bioductory system and mobilize them back to normal. Unfortunately, the mind does not enjoy complete dominance over an ailing brain. If it did there would be no pain, no chronic illness, no death.

Therefore, it is naïve to believe that by a simple wish to be well, the dreaded chronic illness process can be reversed or repealed. Mental placebos have no permanent curative powers over the deteriorating brain, despite the fact that they can appear successful in the short-term after their initial application. Mind action cannot, alone and by itself, remove the cause of chronic brain deterioration which installs the chronic illness process.

The mind can only control the brain to a limited extent. It can for instance determine the way in which a baseball is thrown, a piano is played, and the way work can be done to avoid undue strain on a chronically ill body.

People may safely, even profitably, ignore acute health problems. The leg lost in battle or a car smash or the wages lost at the racetrack are best forgotten as the person concerned endeavors to rise above the setback. But chronic health problems flowing from a chronically deteriorating brain will not go away when ignored, banished by will, or treated with intellectual rapture.

The physician may safely advise his patient to mentally repudiate problems of an acute genesis, for the cause will soon dissipate; but only the charlatan treats chronic problems by telling his patient to will them away.

Very often during the chronic illness process, the mind senses the remission period which customarily follows an exacerbation of an illness. If the mind then commands the body to be well, some apparent and temporary success will be achieved.

Of course, it is always possible to learn to exercise heroic amounts of willpower and disregard the illness. This does not constitute a cure and no self-respecting physician will prescribe such devices as a major or minor thrust of his therapy. Encapsulating symptoms of chronic disorders in a mental cocoon and then rejecting them or stoically and doggedly rising above them is definitely not a proper therapy. For the deadly chronic illness process proceeds relentlessly, and soonor or later exacts its toll on its unsuspecting victim.

It is important to emphasize that, when the chronic brain condition is reversed by Pleneurethical measures, the person often feels that he can now be well simply by an exercise of will or through the power of decision. It is at this point that the person has recognized the recovery process in his or her own consciousness. Actually, the recovery process had been instigated some time earlier by the Pleneurethical restructuring process, and when brain capability was restored sufficiently it became apparent to the mind of the sufferer that health was in immediate grasp.

As the recovery process gains momentum feelings of guilt are also effortlessly abated. Chronic guilt is part of the syndrome accompanying chronic brain depleneurization. Sufferers often feel they are being punished by some unknown but formidable and relentless force, such as a god or evil spirit. (A chapter on guilt appears in volume 5 of *Pleneurethic.*)

PART 4

Mentality commences with the inception of fetal life and ceases at death.

In the beginning the mind reposes adjacent to the brain, but there is virtually no intelligence passing to or from either agency. As the individual matures, the mentality flowers into a structure of incredible complexity.

Mentality is that part of the mind structured by the interplay of brain activity and mind capability. It is a product of both the physical world and the realm from whence mind springs.

The mind is not generated by the brain but mentality, in part, is. Mind knows the material world through the window provided by the physical structure of the brain and the design of the brain limits the frame and clarity of mentality for that individual.

The mind spreads across the total expanse of the brain, working with it in accordance with the latter's structural dimension, both micro and macro.

The infrallect operates primarily below the level of the threshold of ordinary intellectual consciousness. It is associated with that part of the brain's activity that presides over the visceral and vascular segments of the body. It coordinates the activity of the digestive, circulatory, secretory, and reproductive systems and even supervises certain housekeeping chores connected with the operation and maintenance of the central neural system itself.

The infraconsciousness is unilaterally intent on survival. It is selfish to the fullest extent and will seek to preserve the existence of the body for which it is responsible at all odds. It is materialistic with roots deep in the organic wealth of the physical body.

By contrast, the ultraconsciousness, or ultrallect, is all things the infrallect is not. If the infraconsciousness loudly and blindly demands wine, beef, sex, and selfish body love, it is the ultra-consciousness that softly and just as blindly pleads for universal love, survival of mankind, kindness to all living creatures, and empathy with all things living or inert.

The ultrallect is the immediate inspirational source of our ethical and moral nature. The ultrallect bestows upon us what innate regard we have for the rights of others. The small area of the ultrallect that merges with the intellectual consciousness produces spontaneous universal ethical insights and solution of complex ethical and moral problems in a manner that often seems intuitive. This small area of comingling of the intellect and ultrallect generates recognition of those uncommon things referred to as moral guidance, inspiration, and ethical revelation.

The ultrallect illuminates our psyche with thoughts of charity, steadfast pure love, and devoted service to mankind.

Almost everyone experiences some degree of awareness of the ultrallect during quiet and peaceful periods of inner calm. Some individuals seem automatically endowed with considerable aware-ness of the marginal fringes of the ultrallect. This enables such persons to occupy positions of great ethical significance.

Between these two realms of consciousness—the infrallect and the ultrallect—lies a vast mental domain that Pleneurethic terms *intellectual consciousness* or *intellect*. It is that sector of the mentality devoted to ordinary conscious activity and thought. The intellectual consciousness is the source of enjoyment and much satisfaction, if not downright delight, to ourselves and those about us. It is also capable of inflicting cruel abuse when malstructured. Malstructure of the intellect installs acute tension on brain tissues. For this reason we must look closely at the intellectual consciousness and structure of the mentality.

In one sense the intellect may be seen as a living, calculating machine or biological computer. Briefly, the intellectual conscious-ness must recognize, formulate, coordinate, and execute plans to carry out its own estimate of any situation and at the same time entertain influence of the infrallect and ultrallect. To insure formulation of efficient, effective and socially acceptable plans, the intellectual consciousness must be aware of such things as laws, social customs, economic devices, financial principles, negotiable instruments, geography, history, modes of transportation, and methods of communication.

The intellectual consciousness recognizes the existence of the marginal fringes of both the infrallect and ultrallect. It is also cognizant of events outside the body reported by special sensory organs. The intellect develops standard beliefs about its environment and compares new events with these beliefs to determine a course of action.

As choices become more complex, work of the intellect becomes more difficult. Proper solutions to life's problems yield mental happiness, contentment, serenity, and intellectual security. The intellectual consciousness that does not develop proper solutions to problems creates acute mental stress and cerebellar turmoil.

The total task of the intellectual consciousness is indeed of formidable proportions.

The infrallect, ultrallect, and intellect are not discrete, separate, isolated entities. Each partakes of a portion of its neighboring segment. Each encroaches upon the territory of the other and none is mutually exclusive. If a major change occurs in one, the other two are also modified to a lesser degree.

The intellectual mentality may be approached from the categories of function, structure, and content.

The function of the intellect pertains to the inborn manner in which it operates. No one can teach the intellectual mentality to function as a mind any more than we can verbally instruct the liver in performance of its duties of a chemical nature.

The intellect functions when it scans its own content for data and converts it to practical use. It functions when it draws meaningful interrelationships from current or past data and uses this material to solve problems.

The actual mechanics of mind function is imponderable.

Coaching and tutoring may add content to the intellect, but cannot instill ability to function.

Function is such that it can reflect upon itself. The intellect is aware of itself and can evaluate its capabilities as well as the capabilities of the other two segmented attributes—the infrallect and ultrallect. It can restructure its thought content within limits, increase the intellectual mental content through learning efforts, and redeploy itself structurally within limits.

But the intellectual mentality must have possessed the innate or inherent capability of function from the beginning. It can be stimulated, it can be encouraged, but if basic capability is absent at birth, it cannot be created.

The relative vigor or weakness of the intellect in dealing with worldly affairs is controlled to some degree by physiological factors. It functions feverishly and sluggishly in the brain deteriorating through protracted chronic illness. It functions normally when all supportive biological systems are at optimum.

Thus, despite the fact that inherent functional capability of the intellect is set by genetic factors, Pleneurethic practices can bring it to full functional potential by optimizing cerebellar capability.

Structure of the mentality refers to self-adopted beliefs, personal philosophy of life, firmly held desires, basic wishes, and ideas that control the direction of thought and much of our overt behavior. Intellectual mentality is structured on the basis of the things we desire to accomplish and by the desire to avoid certain things. Thus, we desire to survive; we desire to avoid destruction.

It is structured from desires learned and from decisions made to advance or retreat from ideational goals. These may be views, dogma, or theories, as well as material objects. Decisions that become habitual are the essence of intellectual structure. The intellect is free to the degree that it will shift its ideational range.

Thought structure results from a value judgment and often carries an emotional charge received through conditioning and attachment of items of content. A thought structure is relatively unproductive until it becomes entangled with content, which it polarizes about itself.

All other things being equal, the thought structure capable of flexing adaptatively with the pressure of changing events is better than a crystallized and immobile structure.

An individual's intellectual content is composed of those specific items, things, or abstractions he has observed, learned, or experienced. Our mental content is made up of the great mass of perceived observations that we have recorded in our memory.

The specific content of an average mature intellect is unbelievably vast. It may be recorded deep in our memory and be difficult to recall or it may be fresh content on the surface of our memory. The ability to remember does not affect the nature of content.

Mental content in itself is neutral structurally, but it is capable of being polarized. Thus, some content may be drawn to the positive structural poles of those things we desire to have; or the content may be drawn to the negative poles of those things we desire to reject or avoid.

Diseases of the mentality, which are chronic in nature, are best treated by restoring the physical brain to optimum performance. Acute problems of the intellect, created by mental malstructure, are best treated through verbalization on the intellectual level. Treatment on the physical plane may or may not be indicated.

Only the intellect functions in terms of words or concrete pictures. The ultrallect and infrallect deal in sensations and urges.

The intellectual and ultrallectual components of the human being are markedly different.

Whereas the intellectual mentality is inclined to be a law unto itself, placing self-survival first, the spiritual or ultrallectual, when accepted and acted upon, redirects the path of the individual on an ethically higher and more permanently satisfying path.

Selecting one's basic moral direction is the grand work of life, according to Pleneurethical philosophy.

There is no original sin other than the personal sin of freely choosing and following an improper, nonethical course.

PART 5

The chronic anxiety syndrome is a very important discovery of Pleneurethic. Let us now reexamine this phenomenon to fix it more deeply in our mentality.

Chronic anxiety is nature's warning signal of bioductory distortion and disorder as it pathologically stresses the central neurological tissue.

If the neurological cause of chronic anxiety is not abated, loss of confidence and eroded optimism, together with more serious psychological and physiological disorders, will manifest themselves.

Mental and physical illness of a chronic nature accompany each other. But one is not the direct cause of the other as psychosomaticists would have us believe.

Somatic cells and brain nerve cells are on opposite ends of all spinal cord nerve tracts. In chronic illness, mental problems do not cause body tissues to break down nor does chronic body tissue disease directly cause chronic mental illness. Instead, major groupings of spinal cord nerve tracts and even the inferior portion of the medulla oblongata are injured in asymmetrically disordered sections of the bioductory system. These are located between peripherally associated somatic body tissues and central nerve cells in the brain.

As a result of chronic nerve tract pathology, the problem spreads both ways. It patterns out into the body tissues through peripheral nerves. It also retreats along the irritated nerve tracts into the brain cells to cause a real and profound cerebellar disturbance leading to the chronic illness process.

The human brain represents around 3 percent of the total weight of the body in the average person. Yet it requires 25 percent of the total blood supply to provide it with sufficient oxygen and nutriment.

Although brain cells accomplish no physical labor, they aid in mentation.

Thinking is hard work.

It involves such activity as perceiving, interpreting, recalling, solving problems, establishing standards, developing life goals, monitoring activity, evaluating failure, devising alternate modes of behavior, reflecting, concentrating, contemplating, meditating, imagining, determining fact from fantasy, directing sleep rhythm, and setting sexual patterns.

Neurological cellular tissues in the brain preside over the

development, operation, and maintenance of the physical body. They receive sensory messages from all operating tissues and organs. They correlate the messages, determine courses of organic action, formulate orders, and transmit them to nerve tracts for relay to appropriate somatic tissues.

And brain cells have at least one other activity that supersedes all others. They must accept responsibility for the survival of the trillions of other specialized operating cells that, grouped together, form the human domain under the aegis of the brain.

To accomplish this, the brain cells must be vigilant to that which menaces the safety of somatic tissue.

One of the alertive signs is pain.

The greatest number of pain-sensitive nerve terminal fibers are located in the skin, on the exterior surfaces of bones, and on the coverings of organs.

The grand design of Nature to provide this warning system was masterfully executed. However, she overlooked one thing.

She neglected to supply the neural system with a method of determining the exact location of trauma along the surface of major tracts of the neural system itself.

There are few sensory terminal fibers stationed along the extensive surface of a nerve tract. Nor is there anything to elicit a warning of danger to a nerve tract if injury strikes chronically inside a major section of the bioductory system. No lasting pain is reported—only a vague feeling of intense and unremitting anxiety.

The true source of the trauma and resulting chronic apprehension remains nebulous and unresolved if the afflicted person relies solely on his own sensory perception.

According to Pleneurethic philosophy, anxiety (acute or chronic) is nature's way of advising an individual something is inimically amiss. When the welfare of the person is being menaced, anxiety will persist until the danger is abated or understood. When a satisfactory course of action has been adopted and the threat subsides, the anxiety will dissipate with a feeling of relief.

Sources of danger may be open and direct or indirect and covert.

Direct trauma from a sharp object will elicit a consciousness of pain on sensory nerve endings. If someone threatens us with a knife or if we must walk barefoot in the dark through an area infested by snakes or broken glass, we are acutely anxious and apprehensive. Acute anxiety is the normal result in both cases.

But there is another type of anxiety that, prior to Pleneurethic, was thought to be abnormal and baseless—abnormal because it existed, so it was believed, for no reason other than a perverse distortion of imagination.

Pleneurethic believes that chronic anxiety sufferers are victims of direct attack upon the survival of their brains. Traumatically malpositioned areas of the osseous bioductory system are rending or stifling major nerve tracts as, for instance, the spinal cord or inferior aspect of the medulla oblongata.

Confidence is lost as vital brain capacity diminishes. The individual is intensely and chronically anxious but is unable to assign a definite cause for his problem.

Chronic anxiety seldom occurs alone. It is usually accompanied by a family of related negative emotions that form a syndrome.

When such chronic anxiety is elicited by suboccipital, cervical, and upper thoracic bioductory disorder, there also will be chronic tension, emotional instability, apprehension, worry, sleeplessness, loss of confidence, loss of self-respect, depression, intense insecurity, suspicion, despair, resentment, and in final stages, apathy. As the major bioductory trauma worsens and anxiety deepens, we may witness increasing degrees of disorientation, hallucination, mental confusion, nightmares, and even mental incapacitation.

The chronically anxious person is emotionally disturbed by relatively trivial external events. He is not master of his emotions. They are definitely master of him. The depression deepens into apathy as the central neural insufficiency worsens and the disordered bioductories consolidate in malposition.

Hostility and aggression frequently become companion symptoms of some chronic anxiety patients. We find anger, hostility, and hatefully aggressive acts to be out of proportion to the external event that triggered these emotional outbursts.

Such patients are walking bundles of temperamental explosives.

They feel permanent, intense emotions of anger and aggression toward everything, themselves included. At the slightest real or imagined provocation, the thin wall of inhibition is ruptured and hostility breaks forth.

Hypersensitivity also occurs in varying degrees of severity.

Such condition is predictable in view of the constant and unabated spinal cord assault and brain injury from improperly functioning bioductories. Any additional psychological frustration to the afflicted person, no matter how small, in his private day-to-day routine, is enough to precipitate a seemingly exaggerated response.

Trauma in spinal cord and brain often causes deterioration in the individual's ability to perform normal duties. Inability to conduct one's affairs brings self-criticism, insecurity, and leads to loss of confidence. As trauma destroys professional capability and erodes one's social grace, the sufferer senses his loss keenly.

And finally, the chronic anxiety syndrome may bring resentment—deep, intense resentment generated by the manner in which the individual feels his life has been maliciously mishandled by fate.

The basic cause of chronic anxiety, at times, may be reinforced by other factors.

As peripheral somatic tissues and organs degenerate in function and structure from lack of neurological communications, they liberate toxins. Not all this toxin is immediately neutralized or eliminated. As the toxic level in the blood rises, the brain becomes increasingly saturated with it. This contributes to intensification of the preexisting deleterious neural condition. Thus, biomechanical irritation of brain cells due to direct nerve tract trauma is now reinforced circuitously by the caustic action of toxins from deteriorating organic function.

A second manner in which reinforcement of preexisting chronic neurological pathology is conveyed to the brain is through interference with Suri's Tract (the name given by Pleneurethic to a nerve system that originates in the brain, descends the spinal cord to emerge in the upper thoracic area, and proceeds along the sides of the vertebral column of the neck and controls the flow of arterial blood to the neck, head, face, and brain), which controls the flow of blood to the brain.

If arterial action to the brain is impaired, the brain will experience varying degrees of suffocation, chronic malnutrition, and restricted waste removal services following vascular constriction.

Total suffocation, occasional result of a severe accident, will completely destroy brain tissue. Partial cerebral suffocation will yield immediate and intense feelings of anxiety along with physical symptoms ranging from arthritis to paralysis.

Temporary cerebellar suffocation sometimes brings acute hallucination, along with acute anxiety.

Hallucination, along with fantasy and illusion, is a condition of mental activity often associated with chronic anxiety.

Fantasies are simply mental images unconnected with reality. Everyone has periods of lapsing into fantasy, children more than adults. It may be regarded as a form of mental relaxation, an avenue for temporary withdrawal from the realities of the world. Fantasy is normal if the individual recognizes its make-believe qualities.

Illusions can also be more or less normal if they occur nonhabitually. Sense receptors of afferent nerves receive an actual stimulation in cases of illusion, but the mental interpretation of these stimuli is incorrect.

Hallucinations occur when the individual engages in fantasy but mistakenly believes his mental wanderings to be of real substance. The hallucinated individual receives no actual external stimuli, but through mental confusion and bastard automatic brain excitation actually believes he perceives a real event and responds accordingly.

Hallucination can occur under conditions of extreme fatigue, a prolonged starvation period, or heavy neural stress leading to neural insufficiency and exhaustion.

Most chronic anxiety sufferers experience rapid relief from Pleneurethical care.

Relief comes in two stages—the first, a result of the patient's understanding of the true source of his trouble; the second, some days or weeks later, as the burden of major neural disorder is reversed and removed by restructuring procedures.

Mental illness is perhaps the greatest incapacitator in the United States. At least one person out of every hundred is destined to spend some portion of his or her life in a mental institution. These statistics are sobering indeed, but their statistical dimensions are even more shocking when we reflect that these figures refer to the more advanced cases of mental instability.

Pleneurethic contends that many chronic anxiety cases along with accompanying physical symptoms of heart attack and lung disorders can be brought to normal through restoration of brain integrity.

Drug preparations are often recognized in pharmacy as treatment for chronic depression, anxiety, and tension. In the Pleneurethic view, drugs constitute only temporary treatment at best. They are never a cure. The neurological cause of the chronic trouble must be corrected structurally.

Drugs may replace alcohol, marijuana, or religious resignation as a self-help treatment for chronic tension, but drugs often tend to be addictive and are perhaps more harmful than the measures they replace.

Chronic anxiety is one manifestation of the inner energy crisis. Pleneurethic corrects and reverses the cause of this inner energy crisis that creates such havoc with humankind.

PART 6

Let us now examine the subject of dreams and nightmares and their relationships to brain tension a little more deeply. This important Pleneurethical discovery was heralded as the breakthrough of the century by *Saga Magazine* some years back.

Freud, giant of psychology, believed dreams to be of psychological genesis, resulting from hostile desire, repressed wish, or similar psychological mechanism resident in the mind alone. Consequently, he endeavored to piece the mystery of dreams by mental avenues exclusively.

Pleneurethic advances the belief that dreams and nightmares

result from a leveling of cerebellar tissue stress and tension that was previously induced either acutely and psychologically by the mind, or chronically and neurophysiologically by injury and the ensuing illness.

Dreams are a natural process of reducing cerebellar stress and depolarizing content. Excessive intellectual structuring during the day reduces functional efficiency of the central neural system. As normal destructuring takes place during sleep, dreams may occur. They are the natural result of large quantities of psychological content resuming normal polarity.

Daydreaming is also a natural phenomenon. Normal amounts are even beneficial in that daydreaming is akin to night dreaming in reducing cerebellar tensions. Dreams, during sleep, help to level off excess polarity of thought and diminish cerebellar stress generated during the waking hours. Day dreaming may accomplish the same purpose.

When daydreaming interferes with mobilization and productive expenditure of mental discipline, then it should be curtailed. Harm comes if it is permitted to replace necessary accomplishment.

In the sleeping dream state the intellect functions at random, using whatever content is most readily available to account for cerebellar stresses present. The mental operations are undisciplined, hence follow the course of least resistance. Large amounts of content reduce their polarity charge and subside into the neural intellectual content reservoir. In contrast, during periods of wakefulness, mental operations are disciplined, often through compulsion, by the day's events.

The normal dream is produced by brain tension involving *intellectual* activity of preceding days. The nightmare is produced by brain trauma and tension resulting from *mechanical* and *physical* injury to the bioductory system registered on a nonverbal level.

Dreams may be pleasant and placid. Such dreams relate closely to episodes occurring or witnessed in days before the dream and are capable of being expressed on a verbal level. Dreams may also be unpleasant yet still relate to disturbing psychological situations of preceding days. Such dreams are acute, of mental genesis, and are the result of psychologically disagreeable events.

Normally, the body during sleep automatically reduces intellectually generated brain stress that accumulates in brain tissue and is retained until dissipated or removed.

However, stress may come not only from traumatic intellectual events but from mechanical trauma in the central neural system, from poisons consumed by mouth, through the skin or lungs, or from toxins generated within the body by malfunctioning, degenerating, or chemically pathological tissue.

As the body relaxes in supine position, the brain also relaxes. It no longer has the duty of maintaining the body upright or moving it meaningfully.

But when the structural and mechanical integrity of the bioductory system has been destroyed, wholly or in part, the central neurological system does not shed its level of chronic stress during repose.

The result? Nightmares.

Thus, nightmares may reflect accidents that destroyed bioductory structural symmetry many years before, even as far back as birth with use, possibly, of maldelivery techniques.

Recurring nightmares from chronic brain trauma are not amenable to verbal approach but require physical correction of the cause of the trauma—usually a torsion of traumatic proportions in the suboccipital or cervical sectors of the bioductory system.

Nightmare themes are bizarre and hectic because the mind finds it difficult to impute a suitable verbal or social interpretation for chronically violent, mechanically induced brain turbulence of a subverbal, nonintellectual nature.

Dreams and nightmares reflect the condition of our mentality and neural system. The fortunate person who enjoys freedom from neuralosis or intellectosis will seldom be troubled by bothersome dreams or nightmares because the brain relaxes easily. Conversely, the person suffering from severe neuralosis, especially in later terminal years, will be harassed by dreams approaching nightmare proportions because the brain tissues continue to receive low-grade, spurious excitations. Deep restful sleep will also be difficult.

Pleneurethic sees no basic difference between the chronic

anxiety syndrome characterized by the sufferer of severe bioductory trauma and the nightmarish dreams that unrelentingly plague the chronically ill person. They are both a product of chronic mental tension evoked by brain trauma from unabating mechanical harassment of the bioductories.

In a state in which we are clearly and healthfully awake, mental pictures drawn from neurological receptors are accurate indeed—especially in the normally mature person.

When we are asleep the monitoring mind endeavors to compose scenes corresponding to lingering traces of neurological tension patterns. In the sleep state the consciousness is not bound by the same standards of evaluation established by the healthy wakeful consciousness. Wildly incredible nightmares may be one result of the mind's misinterpretation of the true message of chronic brain trauma.

As the neuralosis worsens, the sufferer may have dreams relating symbolically to his ailment. He may dream of being hit on the head with a bat, shot in the head with a pistol, or of falling apart. None of these dream assignations is accurate. They merely denote a chronic abuse to cerebellar tissues of mechanical origin.

Many who claim to analyze bad dreams have been focusing their diagnostic attention on the content of the dream—upon its trivial surface aspects—Pleneurethic asserts.

Chronic nightmares mean the sufferer has a severe neuralosis and continuing neural insufficiency caused by a past physical injury. The treatment is not exploration of one's sexual escapades or feelings of sexual guilt and inadequacy. Rather, it involves abatement of the neuralosis by restoring bioduct mobility in order to repleneurize brain tissue.

Pleneurethically speaking, there is marked similarity between the activity of the central neural system in the sleep state and in the awakened state. In both, it is the neural system that is the actual performer. The somatic cells and the tissues are but relatively inert vassals, subordinate to the neural system. If the neural system and its pattern of energy are distorted, so will there be irregularity in both the sleeping dream state and in the individual's capability when awake.

Thus, in sexual intercourse, for instance, it is not the discrete somatic cells of the vagina and penis that are really performing copulation. The cells of these organs, although individually alive from a metabolic standpoint, do not in themselves directly enjoy the sexually erotic situation. Rather, it is the neural system, directly controlling and regulating the act, that receives the copulatory sensation. In the final analysis it is the two neural systems, one with female sexual apparatus and the other with male, which are engaged in physical copulation.

5

BRAIN-CHEMICAL (FOOD) RELATIONSHIP

PART 1

The chemistry of our body is governed by our brain. The effectiveness with which it directs the operation of the organs and glands can be decisive in the health-versus-illness process.

The endocrine system is a regulatory device composed of glands which secrete hormones and chalones directly into the blood stream. But, whereas hormones excite other tissue to activity, chalones depress activity of the tissues which react to them.

The endocrine system has characteristics in common with the brain. The brain can lash out instantaneously to elicit immediate and specific or general reactions throughout the body. The endocrine system, however, evokes a slower, more prolonged, and less specific reaction throughout the body.

Hormone secretions which excite are something like the operation of the sympathetic segment of the involuntary portion of the brain which also excites. The chalones resemble the parasympathetic portion of the brain since they tend to depress the tissues which are excited by hormones or the sympathetic nerves.

The endocrine system, Pleneurethic believes, was developed as a subordinate member of the neural regulatory agency of the body. The system is controlled by the brain, but once the system is set in motion, it controls a number of bodily functions until the effect of its secretions slowly subsides.

The endocrine system conserves the time and energy of the brain, making it easier for the brain to raise our blood pressure for a prolonged period by simply stimulating the secretion of the adrenal gland.

There is, however, one drawback to this arrangement. If the endocrine system gets out of control, it can make a shambles of our somatic house, our emotional composure, our biochemical balance, and our well-being. This happens when the brain and its nerve tracts which carry orders to the endocrine glands are depressed or irritated. The brain then issues fortuitous neurological directives, but sometimes these nerve tracts are strangled in faulty segments of the bioductory system with the result that neurological paralysis curtails all vital communication with the tissue in question.. Thus, the glands may receive unclear and even false orders which inspire them to untimely overactivity, followed by eventual breakdown and total inactivity over a period of years.

The basic chores of the endocrine system are somatically universal, since the duty of these glands is to assist the brain to control our body. These glands produce widespread somatic and psychic effects.

The master gland of the endocrine system appears to be the pituitary. Its secretions have profound influence on all other endocrine gland operations.

The pituitary, also known as the hypophysis gland, occupies a preferential anatomical position in the body. Not only is it protected by being enclosed within the cranium, but it enjoys further protection by resting in a specially designed bony nest, called the sella turcica, of the sphenoid. It is virtually impossible to accidentally injure the pituitary gland without destroying the cranium and the brain in the process.

The pituitary is also protected biochemically: it is centered in a vascular anastamosis formed by two internal carotid and two intervertebral arteries, called the circle of wills. This arrangement ensures a continued supply of blood to the gland. In fact, if any blood gets to the brain, the pituitary will be the first to get it.

The gland is half secretory tissue and half nerve tissue. The origin of the nerve tissue of the pituitary is in the controlling section of the brain.

A final architectural feature which points to the overriding importance of the pituitary is that its bony nest has its own air conditioning system. As we breathe through our nose air circulates at the base of the sella turcica and the pituitary is always kept cool and nonfeverish.

Because of its appearance the pituitary seems to be almost an extension to the hypothalamus. One suspects that it is endowed with the duty of aiding the hypothalamus to carry out its duty of regulating basic functions in our body. Indeed, there is hardly any bodily function that is controlled by the hypothalamus that is not also affected by the various hormones of the pituitary. The pituitary hangs by the infundibulum from the base of the hypothalamus and reinforces, by chemical hormone secretions, the tasks carried out by the hypothalamus through its neural extensions, the sympathetic and parasympathetic nerves.

It secretes a wide variety of fluid substances which either directly affect the development and operation of the body, or affect other endocrine glands and stimulate or retard their secretory activity.

The multiple hormones of the pituitary affect sexual development and operation as well as affecting both psychic and somatic growth and operation. It helps to regulate the metabolism by cells of sugar, water, fat, and protein. It also aids the regulation of body acid, alkaline balance, and so on.

Pleneurethic aids the pituitary if it is chronically disadvantaged. Nasal passages are often blocked from chronic illness which causes the pituitary to become feverish and operate inefficiently. But these passages will often dilate to normal size under Pleneurethical care, thus ensuring a full supply of air to properly cool the pituitary, which affords relief.

Much of this relief is derived from a cooling action on the pituitary as air once again circulates at the bony base of the gland.

Children whose nasal passages are chronically blocked often seem backward in school. Restoration of nasal passages to normal through Pleneurethical procedures will often permit the proper operation of the pituitary. The resulting improvement of child behavior and intellectual attainment can be astonishing.

Pleneurethic also aids the pituitary, along with general assistance to the entire brain, by removing hindrances from Suri's Tract, thereby ensuring an adequate blood supply to the pituitary and to the hypothalamus. General circulation of all fluids is also improved as ventricles are normalized in the brain and spinal cord.

The thyroid gland, an endocrine gland located at the base of the neck below the Adam's apple, is activated partly by secretions from the pituitary gland and partly by neural innervation. The thyroid gland secretes thyroxin, which stimulates cellular metabolism throughout the body, thereby increasing or decreasing the need for food and oxygen. Thyroxin also regulates the growth of a developing body, including the brain, muscles, and bones. Specifically, hyperthyroidism can create a high metabolic rate, exaggerated bone development, blood sugar problems, high blood pressure, water balance problems, problems in the heart and liver, and so on.

Sympathetic stimulation and regulation of the flow of blood to the thyroid is derived from fibers from the inferior, middle, or superior cervical ganglion which are built of fibers arising from the first four or five spinal nerves. The parasympathetic stimulation is from branches of the vagus nerve. Any problem in the controlling section of the brain or first four or five thoracic bioductory segments or spinal cord in the neck may definitely affect the thyroid. If Suri's Tract is affected, a definite thyroid problem may be produced from the general brain deterioration which follows.

The parathyroid glands, near the thyroid gland, control calcium and phosphorous metabolism, absorption of calcium from the bones of the skeleton, calcium and phosphorous content of the urine, and so on.

Should improper brain communication to the parathyroids develop, problems concerning calcium and phosphorous utilization will arise in varying degrees. Chief among these problems are convulsions and tetany because of calcium and phosphorous imbalances in the bloodstream. The upper thoracic, suboccipital, and cervical sections of the bioductory system may be involved in parathyroid problems.

The pancreas, which produces insulin, thereby helping to

control the sugar level of the blood, is another of the endocrine glands. Sympathetic innervation from the brain to the pancreas is by way of the foramen magnum, major cervical and upper thoracic bioducts, and fifth to the ninth thoracic lateral bioducts. Parasympathetic stimulation from the brain is by way of neurological branches through the vagus. Problems in the brain due to chronic distortion in the bioductory system in the region of the fifth to the ninth thoracics or the major bioductory areas superior to this thoracic region may cause difficulty with the pancreas and its secretion of insulin. Indeed, if the neural problem is severe, functional and structural damage to the pancreas may result, followed by inflammation and swelling. Restoration of disordered neurological communication to the pancreas may sometimes permanently overcome severe health problems connected with the pancreas and its deficient production of insulin. The adrenal gland secretes a hormone called epenephrine or adrenalin. Adrenalin's stimulatory activity upon the body is the same as the action of the sympathetic nerves when in operation, except that adrenalin does not produce sweating as the sympathetics do.

A relatively small amount of neurological tissue is required to keep the adrenal glands secreting adrenalin; thereby achieving a widespread and sustained effect throughout the body. The adrenal gland prepares the body to meet the requirements for intense physical activity. Bitter arguments may lead to fighting, so the use of hard words or angry thoughts may be enough to send the adrenal gland into a state of hyperactivity. This psychological device is often unwittingly used by people to stimulate themselves through activation of the flow of adrenalin.

Adrenalin will affect the eyes, as will sympathetic innervation from the superior cervical ganglion. Both achieve their effect by contracting the muscle of muller, thus pushing the eyeball forward, dilating the pupil, and changing the diameter of precapillary sphincters which control the flow of blood to the eye. Adrenalin also affects all the blood vessels of the body and shifts blood from the skin and visceral organs to the skeletal muscles. When the body is fighting, energy is needed in the skeletal muscles. It is an advantage for the skin to be deprived of blood during battle to reduce excessive bleeding from cuts. Adrenalin has a profound effect upon blood pressure and upon the level of the blood sugar, both of which are increased by adrenal gland activity. Adrenalin will also increase the rate of heart beat.

The adrenal gland receives its sympathetic innervation from the brain by way of branches of the spinal nerves which transit the major cervical and upper thoracic bioducts to emerge through the lateral thoracic bioducts. Parasympathetic communication is from the brain by way of the vagus nerve.

Removal of major bioductory system problems of the cervical and upper thoracic area will often improve brain activity and neural control of the adrenal glands. Within a few months of Pleneurethical care, great improvement may be noted in one's memory, emotional state, heart action, appetite, ability to digest meals, and so on. Improved adrenal action will permit blood to return to the viscera so that meals may be digested properly. A state of general excitement and anxiety may be replaced with a more calm attitude. Even the facial expression may change as the muscles of the muller relax to permit the eyeballs to return to a more normal position in the eye socket. Chronic dilation or constriction of the pupils of the eye may also respond to Pleneurethical care. The eye and adrenal function also respond to correcting the upper thoracic bioductories and lower cervical ducts in the vicinity of Suri's Tract.

The adrenal cortex secretes other hormones in addition to adrenalin. These hormones regulate such important body activities as the utilization of protein, use of fat and starch, and the output of salt by the kidneys.

Generally speaking, the activity of the endocrine system is basic to the development and successful operation of our body. Should sections of it become unbalanced through chronic brain problems, the entire body may suffer hardship. It often happens that through accidental injury to the structure of the major and minor bioductories, the entire endocrine system may be functionally discoordinated. The system may be recoordinated by the reestablishment of normal innervation with gratifying consequences.

Restoration of the brain through Pleneurethical measures

means that the arteries and veins and ventricles of the brain and the fluids that flow through them are normalized after this activity has been interfered with by the consequences of a neuralosis. Removal of a neuralosis, especially in the more cephalward regions of the bioductory system, increases the operating efficiency of nerve cells in the brain and their tracts. It also eliminates the chronic undermining drag on brain cell capability presented by the neuralosis, and its direct physical irritation of major groupings of nerve tissue in the spinal cord.

Most of the basic work in transforming food as it appears on the dinner plate into nutrition suitable for human body cells is accomplished in the gastrointestinal tract, a long muscular tube studded with glands, which is responsible for mechanical and chemical digestion of food. Mechanical digestion is commenced in the mouth, where teeth shred and pulverize the food. After dental mastication, food passes into the stomach and intestines where it is subjected to peristaltic action. This action is the squeeezing, rolling, and pushing movement of the muscular walls of the gastrointestinal tract. Peristaltic action continues at a steady pace until remnants of the food mass, not absorbed, have reached the lower end of the large intestine. It is held there awaiting a convenient time and place for release into the outer environment.

Chemical aspects of digestion are very complicated. It is sufficient to say that digestive juices are first secreted and mixed with food in the mouth; additional digestive juices are furnished by the secretory glands in the walls of the stomach and small intestine. Still more juices are delivered to the digesting food mass in the gastrointestinal tract through ducts from the liver and pancreas. A generous amount of digestive juices is required to react upon the many different forms of food in the tract, to ensure proper digestion and to keep it from putrifying or fermenting.

After it has been properly digested in the intestinal tract, the food is absorbed by the walls of the intestine, where it is collected in surrounding veins. These veins conduct the nutriment material from the wall of the intestines to the liver by way of the portal vein for additional chemical handling before delivery to the arterial system.

Neural innervation from the brain to the gastrointestinal tract is by way of the spinal cord and nerve tracts emerging from about the fifth thoracic to the third lumbar bioducts. The upper and middle thoracic levels control the esophagus and stomach, while the lower thoracic and lumbar levels control the operation of the intestines and colon. Parasympathetic innervation is by way of the vagus. If either section of the dual and opposing nerve system operates irregularly, the tract may be thrown out of mechanical or chemical equilibrium. Thus, the food mass in the tract may be moved so rapidly by excessive neural regulation that the food has no time to be digested properly. This would be called diarrhea and could produce body dehydration and severe chemical irritation to the lower portions of the bowel. Conversely, chronic constipation may also result from an imbalance in neural communication with the tract, because the food mass is moved so slowly that excess moisture is absorbed from the food mass residue destined to become feces.

Improper brain control of the gastrointestinal tract may cause chemical difficulties as well as mechanical problems of food movement. Digestive fluids must be added to the gastrointestinal tract at the proper time and in just the correct quantity. If digestive fluids are poured into the tract when no food is present due to disordered neural regulation, the tract may commence to digest itself. If too little digestant is added to the food, it will likely ferment or putrify rather than become material for absorption into the blood. In this way, the quality of the blood is vitally affected by that portion of the neurological system which controls the operation of the gastrointestinal tract.

Not only may mechanical and chemical digestion be degraded by a disordered and pathological brain and peripheral neural system, but all the walls of the gastrointestinal tract itself may degenerate. If excessive degeneration of gastrointestinal tissues is permitted to occur through inadequate neurological communication, the tract will be unable to assimilate nutriment properly. It may break down into open lesions due to a lack of sufficient blood to its walls, especially if it is forced to do excessive work by the consumption of undesirable substances.

The net result of improper brain control of the gastrointestinal tract will be low-quality blood, malnutrition of the body's tissue and organs, and, finally, degeneration of the walls of the tract itself.

The skin, covering the exterior surface of the body, contains sensory nerve terminal fibers, sweat glands and blood vessels, and so on. So proper operation of the skin is of fundamental importance to a person's well-being. Skin is from one to three millimeters thick, which is sufficient to protect the body from minor abrasions and small cuts.

Sensory nerve endings in the skin warn of danger from those things which are likely to cut, burn, or freeze it. Sweat glands help keep the body cool. About 80 to 85 percent of the excess heat of the body is dissipated through the skin. Skin produces Vitamin D on exposure to sunlight and assists in eliminating toxic wastes from the body.

When healthy, the skin is soft, smooth, pliant, elastic, and resistant to harmful forces. Healthy skin has a distinctive color and is not characterized by either palor or excessive flushing. Healthy skin is clear and never mottled. It does not chronically exhibit blemishes, pimples, rashes, or the like. It is not chronically cold, clammy, sweaty, feverish and dry, extra thin and sensitive, loose and hanging, or tough and insensitive. Nor do we find deep lines chronically engraved in normal skin around the head, neck, and face. There is no paralysis of normal skin.

Skin is richly endowed with neurological communication from the brain by nerve tracts which emerge from all of the thoracic and lumbar lateral bioducts. The skin, like other organs, is innervated by those nerve tracts in its vicinity. Thus, the skin of the arms is innervated by branches from the brachial plexus and upper thoracic nerves and the skin of the legs is innervated from the lumbar spinal nerve branches. Skin is unusual in its neural arrangements. It receives no parasympathetic fibers. Rather, the vasodilator and vasoconstrictor fibers are both carried in the sympathetic nerve tracts.

When neural innervation to a particular part of the skin is disrupted, that area of the skin will become prematurely loose, wrinkled, sagging, and pathologically thinner. Blemishes may appear as pimples, rashes, and warts, and the skin may become insensitive with a feeling of numbness or paralysis, reflecting chronic neurological disorder.

Restoration of the neural supply to the skin often brings about a most welcome transformation and rejuvenation. This aspect of Pleneurethical care is most astonishing when it involves restoring the neural supply to the facial tissues. Usually within six months of treatment a marked change can be detected in the facial appearance of those who have been chronically ill. As facial skin and subcutaneous facial muscles receive more vigorous neural stimulation under Pleneurethic management many things happen, all of which make the face more youthful. The skin becomes more alive and more elastic; it tightens and abolishes wrinkles. Muscles underneath the skin become less rigid and more full-bodied, which produces a softer, more youthful facial appearance. This de-aging process occurs with all persons who have suffered premature facial neural deficiency. If bloating is present it will also disappear under Pleneurethical management.

Although unseen, interior coverings of the body are equally as important as the exterior, but in a different way. Body cavities are covered by membranes which also extend and reflect to invest the organs contained in the cavity. Thus, the brain and spinal cord are covered by a three-layered meningeal membrane: the piamater, arachnoid, and dura mater. The heart and great blood vessels are supported and protected by the pericardium; the chest cavity and lungs are covered by pleura; and, finally, the abdominal and pelvic cavity is aided by the existence of the peritoneum, which holds, connects, protects, and invests the contents, including the liver, large and small intestines, pancreas, and so on.

These protective membranes have a fibrous structure giving them sufficient strength to support the weight of the total organs. They are also equipped with serous tissues which secrete a lubricating fluid. This fluid enables the closely packed organic contents of the body cavities to shift, pulse, and move one against the other with no disturbing pain or physiological reaction from abrasive dry surfaces in apposition. These membranes also store fat accumulated by the body.

Health of exterior and interior covering membranes is basically dependent upon uninterrupted communication with the central neural system via the peripheral neural system.

Much pain and illness may also be avoided if internal organs and cavity coverings are kept well lubricated through proper nerve communication. Manufacture of vital biochemical fluids in our body is performed in small individual chemical factories called gland cells. These cells group themselves together to increase the capacity of their output, also facilitating central neurological control.

Simple glands cover a wide sheetlike expanse of tissue area and discharge their product directly to the surface. Millions of gland cells, which line the inner walls of the stomach and small intestine, secrete directly to the inner surface of that tract. The sweat glands also are distributed through the integument and excrete sweat to the surface of the skin.

Racemose glands, which form colonies of individual gland cells, organize themselves so that their output may be collected in tubules and released at a specific point through a larger gland tube or duct. The pancreas and salivary glands are good examples of racemose glands. In addition to the type of glands known as ducted glands there are the ductless glands, which secrete directly into the bloodstream.

All glands are invariably supplied with a rich capillary network of blood vessels. These vascular capillaries form a nutritive bed in which the gland cells reside and from which the gland cells extract materials to compose their biochemical output. Some types of gland cells merely select material from the surrounding blood supply on a highly discriminatory basis and release it through a duct or on a surface of tissue expanse. Other types of gland cells carefully select various materials from the blood and synthesize these into a new fluid which will be useful to the body.

Both the activity of the glands and the richness of their mine field, the quantity of blood in the vascular bed, is influenced by the brain through its peripheral neurological system. The pituitary, however, is not dependent upon any portion of the peripheral neural system for direct control.

If a certain control center in the brain decides to shut down the operations of a specific gland either directly or indirectly, it can do so simply by contracting the precapillary sphincters which control the flow of blood to the gland's capillary bed. Through this method of opening or closing a capillary bed to the flow of fresh blood, the brain and its nerves influence the activity of such glands as the adrenal, salivary, and sweat, among others. Should any section of the brain become chronically depressed or destabilized, blood flow to the associated gland or muscle will be chronically influenced. Chronic disease results. Initially, the chronic influence may cause the gland to be hyperactive, later—over the years—the gland may become hypoactive, and totally inactive in final stages.

Glands either excrete or secrete biological substances. Excretions are poisonous metabolic waste products which must be eliminated from the body. Secretions are useful materials which are retained within the body to directly aid and assist efficient body operation.

Secretions consist of such things as lubricating fluids to prevent abrasion of certain tissues or eliminate friction in joints of the body. Other biological secretions aid in the digestion of food, stimulation of body tissues to prolonged action, restriction of activity of body tissues, and the counteraction of the effects of other secretions or fluids. Glandular secretions from the reproductive glands are of course required for the survival of the race.

Proper operation of excretory gland tissue is necessary to prevent the accumulation of excess poisons within the circulatory system of the body. Poisons which are sealed off in the tissue spaces and do not reach the circulatory system cannot be excreted. Such poisonous areas may kill our body simply by spreading and enlarging their area of destruction. Neighboring tissues are consumed by contact through fulmination.

One of the chief organs of excretion is the skin, followed by the lungs, kidneys, and mucous membranes of the small intestine.

Skin contains more than two million sweat glands, which expel several quarts of liquid a day under urgent necessity. Some portions of skin are more heavily endowed with sweat glands than others. Sweating can be provoked by a high external temperature, high external humidity, and physical exertion, but it is often a product of pathological neural influence due to a brain upset. Sweat is important to the body from an excretory stand-point because it contains large amounts of urea. Should our skin fail to function because it has been burned, death may rapidly result from excess accumulations of uric acid concentrations in the body. Should our skin operate inefficiently through improper brain control, the concentration of urea in body tissues may increase perceptibly.

If it were not for the lungs, creatures would be unable to survive the lethal concentration of carbon dioxide remaining in their bodies. Carbon dioxide is the noxious gaseous output of cells burning ogyzen and nutritious fuel to produce heat and working energy. Lungs excrete carbon dioxide as blood passes through the pulmonary passageways.

Lungs receive their sympathetic neurological innervation from the brain through the same basic bioductory pathways as spinal nerve tracts leading to the heart and Suri's Tract. The first four sets of thoracic spinal nerves are concerned with pulmonary activity. Parasympathetic innervation to the lungs is derived from the vagus.

Kidneys filter enormous amounts of blood daily and extract a filtrate, called urea, which would poison and kill the brain were it permitted to remain in concentrated circulation. Kidney action is under the control of the brain and the vagus nerve. The sympathetic component of renal neurological communication is provided mainly by branches from about the tenth, eleventh, and twelfth thoracic spinal nerves. The fifth to the ninth thoracic spinal nerves are also involved but to a lesser degree.

Mucous membranes of the small intestines also excrete a

perceptible amount of mucus and other substances of an undesirable nature. These materials are included in the feces and eliminated from the gastrointestinal tract. Feces themselves are not correctly termed excrement because they are not basically a noxious product of the output of the cells as a result of metabolism.

All organs having an excretory function are controlled by the brain by way of the sympathetic and parasympathetic section of our involuntary peripheral neural system. Should either or both of these neural sections of the brain operate improperly, unequally, excessively, or not at all, we may experience chronic illness from organic malfunctions of varying degrees and patterns. Moreover, the organs themselves may eventually become structurally disordered and finally collapse during one of a predictable series of attacks which inevitably and unpleasantly punctuate the course of all degenerative chronic illnesses. Specific body tissues which are dead or dying due to the absence of local neural stimulation must be taken care of. Surgical removal may be indicated if tissue or organic deterioration is irreversibly advanced. If relatively small areas of tissue death are involved, the body will absorb the dead tissues, harden them into a lump, or convert them into pus which perhaps will produce an opening in the skin and drain away. If the poisonous wastes of the dead tissues are moved into the lymphatic and blood circulatory systems, they can present a definite problem to the excretory organs. This is especially true if the excretory organs involved are also impaired by chronic illness processes.

The central neural system, however, never intentionally closes down the supply of blood to any particular gland or muscle entirely, because a gland or muscle cell is always working at some task. During periods when a gland is not actively engaged in secreting or excreting, it must repair itself and continue to live. The act of living and repairing itself does require a minimum amount of fresh blood, hence the blood supply to a gland is never deliberately curtailed. However, if the brain energy supply to a gland and its blood vessel system is shut down by a disorder in the bioductory system, the gland will not receive sufficient nutriment to remain healthy. The gland may become inflamed and purulent, requiring eventual surgical removal if neural innervation is not restored. It can be restored by Pleneurethical procedures if these are commenced early enough. The condition usually requires the consumption of supplementary hormones, digestive compounds, and the like. These can often be discontinued after the brain communication to a disorderly gland and associated tissue is reestablished and the gland has once again resumed normal operation.

Muscles—either visceral, such as the heart and arteries, or skeletal, such as along the arms or legs or back—may lose up to 75 percent of their mass if they are deprived of proper brain communication. Such a debility leads to severe and chronic health problems. Under Pleneurethical care these muscles may be restored to normal, provided irreversible brain changes have not occurred before treatment is commenced. The specific muscle affected depends upon the pattern of bioductory disorder, and consequent region of the brain most involved in the resulting pathology.

Muscles and valves of the heart are vulnerable to deterioration when the brain system fails to properly service them. Death from heart failure may ensue. This can often be prevented by application of Pleneurethical measures.

PART 2

The subject of nutrition is very important to mental and physical health because food affects blood chemistry in the brain. It is also extremely interesting, but it is very easy for an enthusiastic and devoted individual to overemphasize the significance of diet in the control of chronic illness.

Proper modification of an improper dietary regimen can bring relief from acute health problems which have developed as a result of a faulty diet. It is a mistake to believe that the further adjustment of an already adequate diet can reduce the incidence of chronic illness. Faulty diet is never the cause of chronic illness. It can and often does precipitate acute attacks of discomfort and acute debility. It can also reinforce the severity of a long-standing case of chronic illness. One of the other dangers of a faulty diet is that it can generally cause weakness in the anatomical structure that makes it more vulnerable to traumatic stress arising from accidental injuries. And, finally, a faulty diet may install irreversible brain changes in a fetus or young child.

Because acute dietetic problems are not caused by brain pathology from bioductory disorders, these will improve almost as soon as a proper diet is instituted.

But in cases where there is a chronic neural deficiency the best one can hope to achieve through dietary control is to ensure that there are adequate nutritional ingredients in the food that is consumed; ease the digestive burden by eliminating undesirable foodstuffs; facilitate good digestion by the proper preparation of food; and achieve desirable nutritional combinations.

The best diet is one which supplies all the nutritional requirements of the body and imposes a minimal handling and processing load on the neural and digestive systems.

It is better to eat food which is easily digested than impossible preparations which defy complete digestion no matter how much neurological and digestive attention is given to them. It is also better to avoid eating foods which have poisonous side effects because of the toxins which are either inherent in them or added by commercial processors. Improper foods add to the eliminatory and excretory problems of the body, particularly when it has been overloaded through chronic illness tissue breakdown.

Food alone cannot build permanent health. It can only supply necessary constituents which are needed by the brain to build healthy tissues. But no food, regardless of its quality, can remove the cause of chronic illness. Proper diet will remove the symptoms of malnutrition only where malnutrition results from an improper diet. In cases like this the problem is acute and not of a chronic neurological nature.

There is a difference between acute malnutrition caused by the lack of proper food and chronic malnutrition resulting from improper neurological communication. This is particularly so when the tissues in the gastrointestinal tract and their blood circulatory system are chronically involved. This can cause the structure and the function of the walls of the gastrointestinal tract to deteriorate. When this happens they are unable to: secrete sufficient digestive juices; exert proper peristaltic action; or absorb what little poorly processed food is fit for assimilation into the body.

Chronic malnutrition may also occur when the diet is perfect and the digestion adequate because of a specific neurological irregularity. This irregularity can cause the blood-processing organs to operate improperly. When this happens the quality of the blood is reduced. As a result the body suffers from general malnutrition.

Another form of chronic malnutrition can occur in specific body tissue areas even when the blood is of a high quality due to an excellent diet, proper digestion, efficient assimilation, and effective operation of blood-processing organs. As the blood is of a very good quality the body does not suffer from general malnutrition. But a problem in the brain may prevent the distribution of the blood in a particular part of the vascular system to a specific tissue area. This condition can lead to chronic malnutrition in an area associated with a particular bioductory problem. It can affect the limbs and various organs or a specific section of an organ. The only way that this type of malnutrition can be corrected is by restoring normal neurological influence and blood circulation to the deprived area. This can often be easily accomplished through Pleneurethical methods and the results of the therapy are often astonishing.

It is interesting to note that the vitality and integrity of the healthy neural system is near perfect. Wide deviations from the perfect diet can be experienced with little adverse side effects on health and happiness. But, if there is a definite chronic neural problem, even the most perfect of foods and the most meticulous nutritional control will not bestow total spontaneous and buoyant health.

Pleneurethic prescribes no particular diet. But it recommends a diet that is well balanced with sufficient but not excessive caloric quantity and fibrous bulk. The well-balanced diet contains proper amounts of protein, fats, and carbohydrates. It should also include sufficient fresh products to provide the necessary vitamins, enzymes, and other necessities. Minerals are also exceedingly important and great care should be taken to ensure their presence in adequate amounts.

Food should be eaten only when needed and in pleasant surroundings either alone or in congenial company. Excessive fluids should not be taken with meals because digestion may be forestalled through the dilution of the digestive juices.

Fresh foods should be preferred to canned foods or those containing added chemical preservatives.

Food fads should be avoided, especially if they are extended over long periods of time. An all-meat diet is just as undesirable as an all-citrus diet, or all-nut diet. Foods should be changed from meal to meal, day to day, and season to season if possible.

One of the more appropriate guides to diet as far as natural foods are concerned is taste. People who eat natural foods that taste good with a minimum of processing are seldom far away from a good diet.

The taste idea in selecting a diet, however, does not apply to artificially flavored foods. It is possible for an unscrupulous manufacturer of processed foods to prepare substances which taste good but have little nutritional value. Through additives and artificial flavorings, this type of manufacturer is able to mislead people into believing his product is excellent food. Aiding and abetting these fraudulent practices are misleading information on packaging and clever advertising on television, over the radio, and in the newspapers. This type of product invariably reaps a healthy profit margin for its maker.

The caloric quantity required by people depends upon such things as their sex, age, state of health, work habits, the season of the year, their play routine, height, weight, and build. Sufficient calories should be consumed to hold the weight at the proper level. But it is better to choose a diet with the minimum rather than the maximum number of calories. This places a minimal load on the body and the section of the neural system that controls digestion, the processing and the distribution of food.

Utmost attention should be given to the quality of the calories consumed. Low-quality calories are empty calories. They contain few minerals, perhaps no natural vitamins, insufficient amino acids and other vital substances. Thankfully the advent of fresh frozen foods and modern refrigerated transporting vehicles is causing denaturalizing processes, used to abnormally stabilize food and prevent it from spoiling, to fall into disuse.

The foods to be avoided are those which contain calories empty of vitamins, or calories laced with unnatural, limited-vitality vitamins and false sweeteners made from synthetic derivatives. High-quality, high-vitality foods containing adequate natural vitamins and minerals inherent in the food structure should be chosen wherever possible. Such foods may be more expensive than other foodstuffs on the market, but the extra you pay is the best money you will ever spend on food products.

A diet containing high-quality calories is derived from natural food, grown on rich soil, carefully prepared by expert farmers. These farmers pay strict attention to the adequate use of high-quality fertilizers containing all the required minerals and necessary substances. Because high-quality food requires special handling and distribution procedures it costs more, but the higher cost is more than compensated for by the intrinsic worth of the better food. It is not only highly nutritious but it tastes delicious.

The body needs such specific food items as protein, carbohydrates, and fats. It needs protein mostly for the amino acids that are present in it. The body requires nearly two dozen different kinds of amino acids to build its neurological and muscular components. However, not all protein foods contain all of these essential amino acids. Some foods contain one group of amino acids and other protein foods different ones. Amino acids are available in varying amounts from such sources as fresh vegetables, grain, nuts, milk, cheese, eggs, beans, and the flesh of animals.

Each particular type of amino acid is identical regardless of whether it is obtained from a vegetable or an animal source. However, flesh carries a poisonous substance called urea which may add to an already dangerously high level of urea often present in the blood of chronically ill persons. Moreover, the mineral and vitamin content of some meat is relatively low compared to certain vegetables. Meat also lacks significant quantities of bulk to assist in proper digestion. Therefore, vegetable and grain sources of protein are ideal for chronically ill people. Apart from containing no dangerous urea they often have a very high mineral and vitamin content. Vegetables and grains also have bulk, which aids digestion by promoting peristaltic action. The array of amino acids from vegetable sources is usually not as complete as from some meats, so one should become a nutritional expert in order to be able to use vegetables as an adequate source of amino acids. One should remember that the original source of protein in beef was grain and grass.

It is easier for people in some countries to get their amino acids from flesh rather than from grains, nuts, and beans because of their dietetic habits, past education, and accepted marketing practices. Yet it would be wise for people in these areas who are in marginal health to learn about the protein content of the various vegetables, beans, and grains and eat more of them.

Meat should be freshly cooked rather than preserved by the addition of large quantities of chemicals. If nuts are eaten care should be taken to ensure that they are fresh and not rancid, since rancid oil is toxic to the human system.

As different protein foods contain different structural patterns and quantities of amino acids, one needs to be quite an expert on protein to avoid malnutrition, especially if one intends to eliminate meat altogether from the diet.

Millions of the earth's inhabitants, largely outside of the United States, refuse to eat meat protein on philosophical grounds. Instead, they consume grains, nuts, and beans.

Consider the vegetable-versus-flesh controversy for human beings from the level of the infraconsciousness and ultraconsciousness. The infraconsciousness certainly does not care. It will consume the most easily obtainable. But the ultraconsciousness is associated with universal ethic that advocates love for all living creatures. Love does not include fattening a calf and then killing it for food when nuts and grains are available.

One other significant factor emerges in the controversy of animal-versus-vegetable protein. Agricultural statistics show that ten thousand acres of vegetation will provide better nutrition to more people than will the ten thousand acres used to support cattle or hogs. In years to come the public welfare may be directly concerned with shifting the accent on protein harvest from animal to vegetable sources and from land to sea.

Pleneurethic attempts in no way to influence individuals as to how they should secure their amino acids. It is strictly a matter of personal preference whether they choose their protein in the form of a nut from a tree or shoot it on the run with rifle out on the veldt.

But this fact is important: if meat is eaten it should be freshly cooked. Meat preserved by addition of large quantities of chemicals is not in the best interests of proper nutrition.

The carbohydrate portion of a proper diet provides about 70 percent of the total daily caloric intake. Carbohydrate foods, if chosen carefully, will also supply more than 100 percent of the vitamins, minerals, and amino acids. But if the quality of the carbohydrate sources is disregarded, it is possible to receive almost no minerals, vitamins, or amino acids even though sufficient calories have been consumed. This causes the body to be malnourished from mineral and vitamin deficiencies.

Minerals are essential to the proper operation of the body. Without minerals the bones would become soft, there would be no buffer salts in the bloodstream, the pH level would become erratic, and we would tremble easily from calcium deficiencies. The brain and peripheral neural system needs minerals to help it develop and maintain the somatic structure of the body as well as to work bilaterally with the mind. All things being equal, better quality food has the most usable minerals. In recent years minerals have been overshadowed by attention to vitamins. They are, however, of equal importance if not of more importance than vitamins. The healthy body can manufacture many of its own vitamins. It can never, under any circumstances, create its own minerals. It can only rob them from another part of the body. Under normal circumstances, the daily supply of minerals needed to replace those lost through excretion and sloughing of the tissue and other physical processes is extracted from the daily digested food mass and assimilated into the bloodstream. If the diet does not contain sufficient minerals the body's vitality fades. However, it will return to normal once the proper supply of minerals is contained in the diet. This is, of course, provided that the physical problems were caused through an acute mineral deficiency and if they resulted in no irreversible tissue changes.

There are two opposing views toward the addition of minerals to the diet. These are the mechanistic and the vitalistic views. The mechanists believe they can furnish the correct amount of minerals to the diet through capsules containing finely divided metals prepared in laboratories. The vitalists, on the other hand, believe that this is an offense against the public welfare. They are convinced that minerals, before they can be of real benefit to the body, must be taken from the soil by plants and incorporated into living structure. They say that once metal becomes an ingredient of a living plant or animal it is a true source of mineral food for the human body. Therefore, the vitalists contend that chemists should only make mineral capsules to supplement the diet from minerals extracted and concentrated from living plants and organisms.

The need for minerals in the diet is well known to farmers who have to pay high prices for water. They know that the addition of a few dollars worth of minerals to their land saves on water bills. Plants must have minerals to grow. They get these from water drawn through their root system. The plant continues to draw water containing minerals from the soil through its roots, releasing the excess water through its leaves, until it has acquired sufficient minerals to meet its needs. The amount of water the plant takes is governed by the amount of minerals in the water. Thus, if the mineral content of the water is low the plant must consume greater quantities of water.

Similarly, if the carbohydrates taken in the human diet are low in minerals, the body requires more carbohydrates to get the minerals it needs. People tend to get fat on a diet that is mineral deficient. On a high-calorie, low-mineral diet, the appetite can seem insatiable. Mineral deficiencies in carbohydrate foods usually result directly from poor soil or from commercial refining processes that are designed to prevent loss during storage or to make the food look better. Sparkling white granulated sugar, for instance, contains calories devoid of both minerals and vitamins. The same is true of denatured white wheat flour. Both of these products are monuments to public gullibility, commercial chicanery, and political disinterest in the public welfare.

Foods such as raw brown sugar, fresh ground whole wheat flour, and almost all vegetables grown in good soil, contain calories loaded with minerals.

While the mineral content of carbohydrate food was overlooked for many years, the vitamin content of the carbohydrates has been a subject of intense commercial and popular interest for decades. Vitamin supplements are usually not required when the diet consists of natural foods grown on rich soil. They are necessary where the diet is made up largely of denatured, highly refined foods.

Care should be taken when selecting vitamin supplements. Like minerals, the sources of vitamins are a matter of much argument between the mechanist and vitalist schools of thought. The mechanists believe that vitamins can be synthesized from petroleum products. The vitalists, however, argue that unnatural and synthetic vitamins are of little value to the human system. They claim that as a vitamin is a living thing, vitamin supplements should only be extracted from a plant or animal source.

Pleneurethic takes no hard stand in this argument but tends to favor the vitalistic view.

Many discriminating persons are processing their own carbohydrate food items to ensure freshness, and vitamin and mineral content. Some of these have bought miniature wheat-grinding mills. These are electric stone mills and are not much larger than a kitchen-size electric food mixer.

Unfortunately, great dietary abuse does occur in commercial denaturing of enormous quantities of carbohydrate foods. They are relatively unstable and require special handling for distribution and marketing. In their natural state, or after cracking into such items as whole wheat flour, many of the carbohydrate foods are subject to attack by bacteria and other microorganisms which convert the carbohydrate into a mouldy material unit for human consumption. Therefore, carbohydrates are singled out for treatment to avoid the cost of refrigeration and to circumvent financial losses through premature spoilage. These commercial processes succeed in stabilizing the carbohydrate by turning it into an inert substance which will neither be attacked by insects nor become mouldy. But in the process of embalming it with chemicals or sterilizing it with radiation it is turned into a lifeless and practically useless ersatz material. Fortunately there is no need for a great many people today, who have access to fresh, refrigerated, or fresh frozen commodities, to eat such useless foodstuffs.

Another item which has to be included in the diet is roughage, which aids digestion. Foods containing significant amounts of roughage include celery, lettuce, fruit or vegetable peelings, bran of wheat, and whole oats. Little bulk or roughage is found in meat, fat, oil, gelatin, eggs, and flour from which bran has been removed. The roughage sections of grain food, particularly the exterior coverings, always seem to contain a large amount of minerals. In fact, nearly all of the minerals in a grain of wheat are contained in the bran, which is usually removed and fed to pigs. The germ of the wheat, which contains substantial quantities of vitamins and vital oils necessary to good nutrition, is also removed and either thrown away or else fed to cattle.

Oils and fats are also important to physical health. Unfortunately almost everyone underestimates their prime significance. As a result they are usually the first to be eliminated from the diet by people who want to lose weight. But if oils and fats are persistently eliminated from the diet the body will be unable to function properly. This is because these two items contain significant amounts of fatty acids which are vitally necessary to health. Some oils and fatty substances are more useful than others, which may be positively dangerous. The oils on the danger list are those which have turned rancid or those which have been heated to such a high temperature that their nutritional characteristics have been altered. Other oils on the suspect list are those which have been chemically extracted or are hydrogenated. Hydrogenation stabilizes the oil so that it will not turn rancid. The process, however, stabilizes the oil to such a degree that the body finds it difficult to break it down into useful components.

Chemically extracted vegetable oils have to be separated from their chemical vehicles before they are bottled for sale. This, however, is not easy. And often, even though the chemical used in the process is poisonous, it remains in significant amounts in the oil despite attempts to separate the two. Therefore, vegetable oils which have been extracted through cold pressing are the most healthy. In this process vegetables are forced to yield their oil through mechanical pressure alone without the use of either chemicals or heat. Fortunately most of the oils sold today have been extracted by the cold pressing method. But twenty years ago such oils were used by only a handful of health faddists and naturopathic physicians.

Hundreds of books have been published which give good breakdowns on the quantities of vitamins and minerals which the body requires. They also list various foods which contain them. However, such lists are often unreliable as a true guide because the reader does not know which type of soil the food that was tested was grown in.

Food fads which advocate the consumption of certain foods to cure chronic illness should also be treated with caution. For example, garlic has been widely recommended for the control of such things as flatulence, indigestion, diarrhea, and even high blood pressure. There is no question that garlic can be effective in establishing worthwhile but temporary control over acute digestive and vascular problems. However, garlic will not remove the basic cause of chronic gastrointestinal disorders nor vascular problems. Parenthetically, the same applies to most medicinal preparations. They offer only temporary relief for chronic conditions by covering over, easing, or obscuring the symptoms without removing the cause of the complaint.

Under conditions of severe and chronic brain attenuation a temporary reduction of food is often desirable. The time to consume substantial amounts of vital food is when one is feeling well. No harm can come from missing a few full meals in some cases of somatic emergency. In some instances the brain energy required to supervise the digestion of a full meal may be more usefully employed in other precincts of somatic organization. But the treatment of chronic illness by permanent reduction of food below a certain level of intake eventually brings its own complications and terminal events exert themselves rapidly.

Chronic brain attenuation of a general nature and a desire to eat sweet things often occur together. General brain depletion adversely affects the entire body. Conservation of neural energy may be employed on a short-term basis by consuming sweets. Nutriment in this form is immediately available as energy to the body with a minimum of neural and digestive effort. Such a use of sweet things is beneficial if the person realizes the physiological philosophy of the practice and takes steps to receive proper neurological therapy at the earliest practical time.

People sometimes neglect to reduce the amount of food they eat with advancing years when their caloric requirements are less. By doing this they overburden the digestive and vascular systems and those segments of the neural system responsible for controlling them.

There is one final point that should be mentioned in connection with nutrition. Proper nutrition not only brings rewards because of the good things consumed but also because of the improper things avoided. The person who begins to eat properly stops uphealthy dietetic practices. Such a person will refrain from overeating, or untimely consumption of food, no matter how nutritious. He will avoid alcohol, heavy greases, overcooking, and unclean and hopeless combinations of indigestible food. He will avoid high spices, improperly preserved foods, and low-quality commodities which impose a heavy load on the regulative capacity of the brain. The neural system must work overtime to supervise the digestion, assimilation, processing, and excretion of useless or harmful substances ignorantly eaten as food. Overburdening of the neural establishment by a faulty diet may hasten the final collapse of a chronically disordered neural system and the human body it is attempting to regulate.

PART 3

In summary, the primary dietetic aim of Pleneurethic is to fulfill the nutritional needs of the brain in adults and children.

The microstructure of the brain of an unborn child is permanently influenced by the diet of its parents, especially the mother. The child and young adult will be healthier physically, and more intelligent, together with having greater emotional stability, if good brain development is encouraged through nutritious food planning. An unbalanced diet because of poor quality food or poisonous intake such as some drugs and alcohol and smoke, alternately starves and intoxicates the brain and harms its microstructure.

This results in substantial loss to the family and the world community, to say nothing of an unnecessary blight upon the self-esteem of the unfortunate individual because of his or her reduced level of competency.

Let us now review the subject of food as it relates to brain.

Inadequate and improper nutritional diets may acutely affect the brain and its sufficiency. This comes not only through the useless work of digesting and processing substandard food but more significantly through failure to provide suitable sustenance.

Improper diet may, indeed, reduce the vigor of the system totally. This does not necessarily take the form of chronic illness but it can bring acute reduction of life potential through poor quality blood from deficient fuel intake.

The result? Malnutrition and substandard brain performance.

Prolonged nutritional deficiencies will precipitate all manner of difficult-to-diagnose problems, including developmental deficiencies of brain in the young.

Simple malnutrition is inadequate or improper consumption of food. Complex or chronic malnutrition is a failure of body tissues to assimilate nutriment despite proper consumption.

The chronic malnutrition that menaces the body when food intake is nutritiously balanced derives from chronic brain condition and neural insufficiencies of digestive organs or distributive systems from neuralosis.

Certain patterns of neuralosis cause a continuing hunger, others a revulsion to food. Persons suffering from the former eat constantly to satisfy an insatiable appetite. This tends to cause a chronic obesity. The other form brings a drastic and habitual curtailment of food and precipitates a chronic frailty bordering on emaciation.

Faulty diet is never the cause of chronic illness, although it can and often does precipitate acute attacks of discomfort and acute debility. Modification of an improper dietary regimen may bring relief from acute nutritional problems that have developed solely as a result of faulty diet. But it is a mistake to believe that further adjustment of an already adequate diet will reduce the incidence of chronic illness.

Pleneurethic considers the best diet to be that which supplies all necessary nutritional requirements of the body and imposes a minimal handling and processing load on neurological and digestive systems.

Food alone cannot build permanent health. Food can only supply necessary constituents that are used by the neural system to build healthy tissues. Proper diet will remove the symptoms of malnutrition only where that malnutrition is a result of improper diet. Hence the problem is acute and not of chronic neurological nature.

The most desirable nutritional condition finds the neural system operating at plenary potential, complemented by a fine diet of highest quality.

Pleneurethic does not prescribe any particular diet.

Food consumption should be well balanced, however, with sufficient, but not excessive, caloric quantity and fibrous bulk. The well-balanced diet contains proper amounts of protein, fats, and carbohydrates. It includes sufficient fresh produce to provide necessary vitamins and enzymes and adequate amounts of minerals.

Fresh foods are to be preferred to canned or chemically preserved. Foods that contain calories empty of vitamins or calories laced with unnatural, limited-vitality vitamins and false sweetening made from synthetic derivatives are to be avoided. High-quality, high-vitality foods containing adequate natural vitamins and minerals inherent in the structure and content of the food are the best choice.

A diet containing high-quality calories is derived from natural food grown in rich soil. Commercially grown food is often tasteless and nearly worthless nutritionally because of high profit commercial practice that sacrifices quality for quantity.

Minerals are essential to proper operation of the body. They help develop the neural system and maintain the somatic structure. Generally speaking, the food with the most usable minerals is the best food.

How best to obtain minerals in the diet?

There are those who believe proper mineralization in the diet can be provided through encapsulating finely divided metals prepared in the laboratory with mortar and pestle. This is strictly a mechanistic point of view.

On the other hand, the vitalists believe that before metals can be of optimum benefit to the body they must first be taken from soil by plants and incorporated in the living structure of that plant.

Once the metal becomes an ingredient of a living plant or animal, it thereby becomes a true source of mineral food for the human body. Such mineral content, they believe, can be encapsulated as dietary supplements but only after it is extracted and concentrated from *living* plants or organisms.

The intelligent reader may draw his own conclusions on the question of vitalism versus mechanism.

Again, in selection of these supplements the mechanists and the vitalists may tangle. The mechanists believe that vitamins can be synthesized from petroleum products in the pharmacist's laboratory. The vitalists offer the counterargument that unnatural and synthetic vitamins are a serious offense against the uninformed and trusting public. They contend petroleum products are for consumption by inanimate machines. A vitamin, they believe, is a living thing that can be properly encapsulated and labeled a vitamin only when it has been concentrated from living vegetable or animal source.

And again, Pleneurethic takes no definite stand on this highly controversial question. However, if there must be a preference, Pleneurethic leans toward the vitalistic side.

Some discriminating people now privately process their own carbohydrate food to insure freshness, vitamin, and mineral content. Miniature electric stone mills, not much larger than electric mixers, are available. In such a machine, high mineral content wheat can be ground at home to provide a fresh supply of unrefined and uncontaminated whole wheat flour.

Roughage is another necessity in the diet.

Without bulk, digestion will be hindered. The food will not move in an orderly manner through the gastrointestinal tract if bulk is absent. Roughage is composed of indigestible and nonabsorbable food fibers and is found in such foods as celery, lettuce, peelings of fruits and vegetables, bran of wheat, and whole oats.

The prime significance of oils and fats in the diet is frequently underestimated. Regrettably, oils are the first to be eliminated from the diet of the would-be reducer. Yet, if oils are persistently eliminated, the body will be unable to function properly and normally. Oils and fats contain significant amounts of fatty acids that are vitally necessary to health. On the other hand, some fatty and oily substances are dangerous. For instance, those that have turned rancid or have been heated to such a high temperature, so that their nutritional characteristics have been altered, pose a danger.

Suspect, too, are those oils that are hydrogenated (stabilized to prevent them from becoming rancid but to such a degree that the body has difficulty splitting them into useful components) and those extracted chemically. In the latter process, the vegetable oils must be separated from their chemical vehicles before they are bottled. The chemical is poisonous and may remain in significant amounts even after separation.

Vegetable oil that has been extracted through cold pressing is the most healthful.

Twenty years ago cold pressed vegetable oils were used only by a few forward-looking people and by naturopathic physicians who were apt to be subjected to ridicule for their practice. Now this oil is sold as a standard shelf item in supermarkets everywhere.

Another idea advanced by naturopathic physicians a quarter of a century ago and now generally accepted by professionals and laymen alike is that of the preferred use of vegetable oils over those derived from animals.

In general, the person who wisely adopts a healthful nutritional regimen will be quick to abolish unhealthful dietetic practices. He will refrain from overeating and from untimely consumption of food no matter how nutritious it may be. He will avoid excessive alcohol, heavy greases, high spices, improperly preserved foods, and low-quality commodities that impose a heavy load on neural regulatory capacity.

The neural system can be overworked in digesting, assimilating, processing, and excreting useless or harmful substances in the diet. Overburdening of the neural establishment by such faulty diet may hasten the final collapse of a chronically disordered brain and the body it is endeavoring to regulate.

6

BRAIN-PHYSICAL RELATIONSHIP

PART 1

In Pleneurethic, the brain is the central factor in much unexplained illness and is the central basis for continued good health.

Much brain disturbance, either passing and acute or more lasting and chronic, is caused by structural distortions, accumulating in the brain. The sources of brain distortions are both internal and external. The brain is subject to demands of the mind and mentality as well as to the press of a worldly environment. It is also closely occupied with the maintenance of the body from which it receives vital support. After the body has nourished the brain, cooled or warmed it, transported it, and provided for reproduction, it can do little else.

A clear, clean, and well-structured brain responds easily to all that is thrust upon it. But, when the brain becomes sodden and destructured from chronic traumatic overburden and chronic undernourishment, it responds erratically and unnaturally—if it responds at all.

Pleneurethic holds that the mind and the body are not the same, as other disciplines proclaim. It contends that the mind and body are separate and that the brain is the special mediating tissue that separates them. The brain is a universal tissue capable of communicating both with mind and body and the external world omnidirectionally. It is vulnerable to accidents which harm the body. Chief among the incidence of such accidents are those to the body's bioductory system.

The bioductory system, a basic anatomical system of the body, plays a leading and usually definitive role in the chronic-illness-

128

versus-health process. It is especially important because of its fundamental and widespread influence on mental and physical health due to its intimate association with the brain.

Pleneurethic was the first school to note the significance of the bioductory system, to give it a name, and to mention it in writing.

The lack of knowledge of the existence and significance of the bioductory system led to the concoction of other theories about the cause of chronic illness over the years. These other theories gained widespread acceptance. However, they have now been proven to be worse than useless because they are misleading.

A new epoch in understanding the brain and in healing chronic illness began with the release of Pleneurethical findings in January, 1965, to the leading scientific institutions throughout the world.

The bioductory system conducts and protects the brain as it directs, regulates, and coordinates all somatic systems of the body. Much of the bioductory system is flexible—within limits. And its proper operation depends on the preservation of free mobility of interconnecting segments. The bioductory system contains and transmits the nerves in much the same manner as the circulatory system funnels the blood, the pulmonary system channels the respiratory gases, and the digestive system mixes and pushes the food along, supplying it with proper juices en route. It surrounds the nerves and forms both osseous and soft tissue ducts through which the nerve tracts pass. The system directly supports, shields, and aids the brain. This is quite obvious when one realizes that all nerves are actually brain tissue extensions.

The bioductory system is physically more extensive than the pulmonary system, more intimately interrelated with the brain (physically speaking) than any other system, and is the system with which the brain system is anatomically coextensive.

The bioductory system starts with the cranium and spinal canal and includes all neural foramina of the cranium, all spinal foramina, and the intervertebral foramina. It also includes all soft tissue tubes which transmit both afferent and efferent nerves of the peripheral brain. The brain itself is always at the mercy of the bioductory system, particularly the osseous portions which the brain laid down early in the life of the individual to protect itself and provide surfaces of attachment for skeletal muscles and so on.

If the bioductory system, especially the central osseous sector, is traumatically maldeployed through some accident it no longer protects the brain. Instead it acts as its slow executioner by altering the supporting physiological systems. The broken and destructured bioductory system absorbs large amounts of brain energy unproductively and hinders the brain in its efforts to restore itself.

The chronically disordered bioductory system is the main source of chronic problems to the brain, during its effort to maintain a proper balance of energy for use by the mind and somatic systems. The chief duty of the bioductory system is to permit the neural system to retain its structural symmetry and integrity while the brain attends to its many affairs. The interior of the bioductory system transmits the brain and its neurological extensions, the exterior provides surfaces of attachment for muscles and ligaments.

Damage to the bioductory system is harmful in several ways. It can destroy the brain itself. The extension of the hind brain, or spinal cord, and its roots may be crushed, even torn in two depending on the extent of injury to the bioductory system. Blood can be cut off from the stricken area of the neural system and in some cases this can lead to a total breakdown of the spinal nerve tracts and spinal cord in the area, thus impairing control of the body and even circulation of blood to the brain. This is especially true if the bioductory problem is in the neck or shoulder area. Or the brain could be disturbed by spinal cord trauma as a result of an accidental injury to the bioductory system.

The brain disturbance can display many characteristics, depending on the area affected. It can range from unconsciousness to headache to hyperirritability and overactivity in the initial stages. Later stages may yield hostility, fear, volatile emotional behavior, restless sleep patterns, dizziness, and nausea. The brain becomes overloaded, destabilized, undermaintained, and depressed as chronic anxiety plagues the sufferer. Under the pressure the memory may deteriorate.

Local trauma to the bioductory system in the immediate area of damage can also cause pain, swelling, stiffness, and, in the final stages, arthritis, ankylosis, and paralysis. The exact nature of the complication depends on the extent and location of the trauma and the way it is attended to or ignored. The nature of any other injuries which may have been incurred to the bioductory system could also determine the course of any future ailment.

As the bioductory system hardens from injury or old age, the nearby spinal muscles deteriorate and weaken. As they do so the rate of degeneration accelerates. All body systems deteriorate according to the pattern of bioductory disorder and regenerate in company with bioductory restoration. Conversely, normal flexibility of the bioductory system fosters physical development.

Harmful distortion in the structure of the bioductory system creates correlative patterns of distortion of pathological dimensions in the brain and throughout the body and mind.

Relating chronic mental and physical illness to chronic brain disorder is unique to Pleneurethic and an important key to the understanding of Pleneurethic. Chronic illnesses are those disorders which, because of chronic brain insufficiency, will not correct themselves automatically with time; medically through pharmaceutical formulations; nutritionally with dietary modifications; athletically through physical exercise; psychotherapeutically through regular psychological analysis and treatment; or through general shotgun-type manipulations of the spine. Chronic disorders will only respond to Pleneurethical correction which reliably restores brain sufficiency by correcting the specific bioductory cause of the brain insufficiency, and considers acute problems which may contribute to the total unproductive load on brain.

Acute disorders heal automatically. Thus, a finger which has been cut will heal automatically. A hand which is mangled will heal automatically, although it may be misshapen unless it has been attended to by a plastic surgeon. However, a hand which is mangled may become a chronic problem and require amputation if the lower cervical bioducts were also severely injured in the accident. In such a case the brain and nerves from the spine which innervate the tissues of the hand will become chronically traumatized in the lower cervical bioducts. As a result the tissues of the hand will suffer from specific brain insufficiency which will establish a chronic condition.

The main difference between chronic and acute disorders is that a chronic condition will not get well by itself because of brain insufficiency. A person cannot correct his own bioductory trauma. Fortunately, acute conditions do not physically impair the fundamental brain sufficiency control system. Because of this an acute condition has the potential to correct itself since nerve damage is not involved nor is brain operation in the bioducts hindered. As a result the acute condition possesses the brain power to automatically repair itself. The chronic condition does not.

Some acute accidents can kill. But in these cases, death is due to the loss of blood from cut blood vessels, asphyxiation, heavy shock, poisoning, and so on. If an accidental death was caused by a massive brain-bioductory collapse occurring through severe trauma, the cause of death was chronic. This is true even if the death occurred in a matter of a few moments, minutes, or hours.

Chronic illness originates from either a general or specific brain insufficiency. It is generated by chronic brain insufficiency created by traumatized, malpostured, hypomobile areas of the bioductory system. Such a condition requires external forces applied by an intelligent operator to relieve it. As we said earlier, chronic illness will not improve by itself automatically, although it will be characterized by cyclic periods of exacerbation and remission, with perhaps gently declivitous plateaus in between. Chronic illness is not a thing of the intellect or of spiritual ethic. It stems from structural trauma of the material body's bioductory system.

Acute illnesses, on the other hand, are all ailments other than those of chronic or of congenital etiology. Acute illnesses may be caused by excesses of all kinds. Food poisoning results in an acute illness. Overeating may lead to acute distress. Worry over a real-life situation may cause acute constitutional illness. The therapy for acute disease is not the restoration of brain bioduct sufficiency, regularity, and posture. Treatment calls for surgery, allopathy, homeopathy, medicine, chiropractic, osteopathy, naturopathy, prayer, laying on of hands, and psychotherapy (which includes all forms of mind) and mental cures.

Pleneurethic holds that congenital illness is neither acute nor chronic. Congenital illness does not result from chronic reductions of brain sufficiency. Congenital ailments, such as missing limbs, are caused through the absence of proper brain structure from the moment of conception. Therefore, these are problems of a genetic nature and fall outside the scope of Pleneurethic.

Improper ways of thinking will never directly disorder brain or bioducts in such a way as to create a chronic insufficiency. However, such mentation, although it may be technically acute, does aggravate whatever chronic problems exist. For this reason, all mental problems which are stubbornly acute will be treated by Pleneurethicists. Moreover, some mental problems are derived from the chronic illness process and are entirely chronic. The Pleneurethicist must be able to accurately discriminate between the various forms of mental problems and disturbances.

In Pleneurethic the physical body is divided into two broad classes of tissue: the somatic body and the brain system. The somatic body includes all nonbrain cells, tissues, and organs. The brain system is comprised of the brain, spinal cord, and peripheral nerves. Mentality exists in addition to the physical body.

Although physical disorders of the bioductory system are the initial and basic cause of chronic illness, both mental and physical, the bioductory disorders in the beginning cause nothing more untoward to the intellectual consciousness of the patient than a backache, neckache, or headache and spinal stiffness. Bioductory disorders cause an inharmonious pattern or neural mechanico chemicoelectrical irregularities which in turn cause progressive deterioration of somatic function, mental function, and breakdown of somatic organs and central brain tissues, with eventual demonstrable lesions and symptoms which cause the patient discomfort.

Thus, the symptoms which bother the patient come from a

series of causes, each successive link veiling its predecessor. It is for this reason that patients have never been able to reveal to doctors the real cause of their chronic suffering. It also explains why chronic sufferers are susceptible to a multitude of different approaches to healing—all ineffective, but plausible, because they ameliorate some of the symptoms, or links in the chain of causes and effects.

Pleneurethic, therefore, does not treat the entire physical body or surface symptoms of suffering, but in the treatment of chronic illness addresses the major part of its operation to the restoration of brain sufficiency by restructuring the bioductory system to normal. This is accomplished with the aim of restoring the normal pattern of brain functional activity and through this send further benefits to all parts of the body which are chronically ill. When the system is normalized the brain is able to reverse and abate the cause of the chronic illness process in the body.

When brain integrity is restored Pleneurethically, organic functions which were previously depressed by the chronic neural degeneration will not improve uneventfully. During the period of regeneration there will be periods of overcompensation followed by periods of undercompensation as the neural system seeks to establish normal equilibrium, both within itself and the peripheral somatic tissues which it governs. Stable tissues and organs of the body which were operating normally before Pleneurethical treatment will remain normal during Pleneurethical care. This means that there will be no reversals or periods of underactivity or overactivity in organic tissues or bodily functions which had not degenerated or become depressed through chronic disorder. Only chronically disordered tissues and organs will exhibit rejuvenative reactions as they respond to Pleneurethical care and faithfully return to stable operation and normal structure.

Some of the rejuvenative indicators are not pleasant, and some patients feel discomfort. Many patients, however, feel no discomfort whatsoever. They simply begin to regain a general feeling of optimistic well-being. Moreover, as the rejuvenation process continues all patients report having more energy, a clearer head, a better memory, and an increased libidinous energy level.

The inability to clearly discriminate acute and chronic illness has handicapped healing, healers, and patients for centuries. In cases of acute illness, the patient points easily to his hurt. In chronic illness the person just feels awful. He has great difficulty in being precise about his chronic complaint for he may have little or no specific pain or ache. The inability to be specific misleads the orthodox healers into jumping to an unfounded conclusion that the ailment is either some highly variable and mysterious form of acute genesis or is of psychological origin and the patient is crazy, hysterical, lying, imagining, malingering, and so on.

Since the sufferer is able to accurately describe the complaint in most instances of acute illness, the doctor insists upon accurate reporting of hurtful symptoms in all cases before he will take complaints seriously. The drug-oriented doctor, not knowing the general difference between manifestations of acute illnesses and those of chronic illnesses, makes a botch of nearly every case of chronic illness he ill-advisedly attempts to treat. He may perform brilliantly on acute cases, but more often than not misses the point completely in chronic cases. Very often in chronic cases, the pharmaceutical physician cannot find a cause of the illness complained of and indeed cannot even find evidence of the illness itself unless the body organs are in an advanced stage of deterioration and a major biological disaster is patently at hand.

While genetic anomalies do not cause chronic illness, chronic illness may cause genetic anomalies. Genetic patterns in germ cells of fathers and mothers may be disturbed because the organic tissues which produce the germ cells or support them after conception are inadequate. Such inadequacies may result from inheritance, radiation, poisonous side effects of drugs, alcohol, industrial poisons, and from Pleneurethic's bioductosis and neuralosis with ensuing neurological insufficiency to the gonads.

Patterns of trauma in the central brain tissues throw correlative patterns of distortion into the mind and soma. These patterns can cast a general depression over the entire body or select isolated tissue areas. It is not unusual for the pattern of chronic illness to be such that the reproductive system becomes incapable of creating a complete germ cell or of sustaining it if conception is achieved. Chronic illness processes are ordinarily quite slow, but in the initial stages the affected somatic region may even be overstimulated. In those cases where the sexual apparatus is affected, the person may be hyperactive sexually for a few years. Then, after a slight fever or rash or discharge in the affected somatic area, it will begin to degenerate. It is in this stage, prior to total sexual incapacity that a defective germ cell is likely to appear.

Congenital deformity may be prevented by Pleneurethical therapy in those cases where chronic illness has forestalled the prospective parents' ability to produce germ cells with proper genetic pattern. In this way Pleneurethic prevents congenital deformity caused by defective genes in a chronically ill person. However, corrective therapy to arrest this likelihood must be begun before the occurrence of a degenerative exacerbation which is capable of destroying any area of brain tissue associated with reproduction. Although congenital deformity is not a form of chronic illness, some chronic degenerative disorders will pre-dispose parents to throw defective germ cells. If the chronic illness is severe and of fairly long standing, flaccid sexual apparatus and lack of interest in copulation may deny introduction of defective germ cells to its mate. If proper introduction is achieved, the defective germ cell may be so inadequate that not even a congenitally deformed fetus will be produced.

Chronic illnesses are variable and not all such illnesses produce similar effects in the mind and in the body. Certain chronic illnesses can cause an alteration in the genetic struc-ture of the sperm or ova cells manufactured in the sexual ap-paratus of the chronically ill person. Once such a deformed cell is produced, conception from it will create a congenital deformity. After the individual with the congenital deformity commences to live, the process of deformity cannot be reversed.

There is an element at play in the armament of the intellectual that hitherto has not been well understood. The very healthy intellectual is courageous, confident, clever, witty, with good memory, and in fine spirits. But also of significant importance, his brain and neural equipment are unhindered by direct irritation of a physical or biochemical nature leading to brain exhaustion and eventual deterioration as in bioductosis.

It is very easy for the "intellectual" being, free from chronic illness, to really believe that only the attitude of intellect is of prime significance in an illness. Because he does not know the utterly disturbing, depressing, and distorting effect of physical bioductosis on brain function and the mentality as well as the soma, he fails to consider the overriding significance of brain trauma when it exists in others not so fortunate as himself. Many unfortunate people who seem substandard or only average suffer not from an improper mental attitude but rather from an enervating neuralosis.

This should not be construed to mean that one cannot be an intellectual and at the same time have a concurrently moderate neuralosis. However, in such cases the intellectual will know he is ill and will continue working in spite of the chronic illness which attends his particular patterns of neuralosis. He will not be able to work effortlessly, nor will he experience the exuberant, irrepressible good mental and physical health enjoyed by the healthy intellectual. Moreover, the neuralotic intellectual will be inclined to exhaust himself at an early age and perhaps perish, become a suicide, or have an involvement with mental institutions.

PART 2

Spine engineering of man was designed for horizontal posture.

Closely note the gross structure of a human vertebra. It was fashioned to be suspended on a horizontal axis—not vertical—suspended horizontally between two arms or forelegs and two hind legs. The bodies of human vertebrae, especially in the lumbar and thoracic regions are heavy in proportion to any other part of the vertebrae—much heavier than the spinous process that is diametrically opposite the body.

If a vertebra is suspended horizontally, the body is heavy enough to cause the vertebra to properly position itself. If a series of vertebrae are suspended horizontally, they will all automatically assume similar positions: i.e., bodies down, spinous processes up. The force of gravity alone accomplishes this.

One might say the fall of man was consummated when he rose up on his hind legs and made arms of the fore. Assumption of the upright posture inaugurated agony, suffering, and hardship, as indeed did the move from a watery environment to that of land.

A multitude of physiological problems arise from faulty posture. Some are the result of accidents that have harmed the anatomical basis for proper stance. Posture begins with carriage—the way we stand—the anatomical relationship of our bioductory segments, their general condition, the sufficiency of our neural establishment.

Abnormal postural characteristics of parents acquired through accidental trauma may often be passed on to children, not by inheritance but simply by the imitative qualities of the young. Thus, the parent with heart or lung trouble due to trauma in the upper thoracic area may influence his child to adopt the same anatomical postural abnormality. Later in life the child, too, may acquire heart and lung problems. In this way, faulty and abnormal posture may be handed down through generations, with family members mistakenly believing its heart and lung weakness to be an inherited internal deficiency beyond their control.

This same principle is also involved in dietary habits and tendencies to certain types of obesity.

Physical exertion will not alone provide solid basis for health any more than mental drill will increase the I.Q. or sharpen basic insight. Each individual inherits a specific neurological potential for stamina, symmetry, and muscular power. A normal amount of physical and mental exertion is all that is required to develop that potential. If an individual fails to perform this normal amount on a day-to-day basis he may become weaker, but this physical weakness is not a form of chronic illness. It simply means his muscular system cannot be called upon suddenly to carry out a work assignment in excess of normal output.

It is also true that one who overexercises to add to his normal muscular development does not create additional health. But the precise ability to overdevelop a muscle means that the neurological system is still operating. Hence, it is in reality a crude test of neurological integrity and capability.

Total inactivity in our living regimen would eventually bring death. Physical exertion and muscular flexion promote circulation of body fluids by squeezing the blood and lymph through valves in veins and lymph ducts. As venous blood and lymph are moved, space is created for more arterial blood carrying food and oxygen to body tissues.

But it is possible to overexert and destroy bioductory system integrity. Excessive exertion and violent exercise may injure the sections of the bioductory system and damage associated nerve tracts leading to the brain, thereby weakening the body in the long run.

Brain capability furnishes the necessary bulwark for sustained health. Thus, avoidance of all things that injure the brain, directly or indirectly, is axiomatic.

Light irritations over a long period of time will damage brain capability just as surely as heavier trauma over a shorter period.

Physical force, not words, directly applied to the body, is the cause of damage to the bioductory system.

Sectors of the system are sometimes collapsed or impaired when the adolescent proudly demonstrates his strength by lifting the rear end of the family auto when it is loaded with girls. They are collapsed when the young football player is tackled from behind by a 200-pounder, or when the infant is grappled and twisted by steel forceps during a difficult birth. Injury may come in skiing accidents, in a dive into water too shallow for cushioning the impact, in an unguarded blow to the head in boxing, or an improper fall in gymnastics.

Abundant statistics reveal the relative age of men and women at death. Women live longer, on the average. The simple basic reason, Pleneurethic contends, is that women seldom abuse their bioductory systems and impair neural sufficiency as often as their brothers.

Physical activity may be divided into three basic levels of exertion, pertaining to insufficient, sufficient, and excessive amounts necessary for optimum health.

The first refers to a range of body movement and activity insufficient to maintain proper physiological function of body tissues and organs. An insufficiency of physical activity leads to acute atrophy of tissues and simple signs of nonchronic illness.

The second level refers to a range and quantity of movement required to keep body tissues and organs operating efficiently. Normal living movements of the average person ordinarily suffice.

The third level refers to additional amounts of unnecessary exertion that may develop large and bulging muscles and may also yield a temporary overabundance of muscular stamina and endurance permitting performance of heavy physical assignments.

Many persons find themselves overexerting their muscular system simply because they have failed to adapt their thinking to advancing age. No middle-aged man wears the same clothes he wore as an adolescent nor does he conduct his social and economic affairs as he once did. The ordinary amount of physical exertion characteristic of normal youth becomes an excessive level of muscle utilization if projected into middle age.

With growing children, greater activity is required to provide an increased flow of blood to developing muscles and tissues. After adolescence, the tissues are fully developed. Normal amounts of exertion are sufficient. With the onset of old age, less movement is required. Muscles are naturally diminishing as our neural capability fades.

What type of physical fitness program does Pleneurethic recommend?

Sports that do not unduly or violently compress or rotate the sections of the bioductory system are best. Swimming, because it extends the body as it is supported horizontally in the water and develops both sides of the body equally, is efficacious. Diving, on the other hand, may injure suboccipital and cervical bioductory regions.

Walking especially in open hilly country is an excellent recreational outlet and provides a way of performing normal living movements that do not overtax or overdevelop the body.

Calisthenics, with the exception of tumbling, acrobatics, and violent forward-bending maneuvers, perhaps provide a more sensible way of securing physical exercise than sports. In general, sports, especially American-style football, are apt to be excessively strenuous and even injurious.

Of all calisthenics, one of the most beneficial is the Chinese system of exercise. Basically, the Chinese exercise coordinates mind and body. Mental concentration is required as the exercise is performed. Physical movements are slow, graceful, and skillfully executed. No great physical exertion is required, hence there is no overdevelopment of muscles. The Chinese method, however, overlooks no movable joint, no skeletal muscle of the body.

Not all Oriental exercises are without criticism. Body yoga is dangerous because many persons, particularly Americans, are stimulated to practice it unsupervised. The most potentially dangerous of all are those movements wherein the weight of the body is inverted. Thus, virtually the entire weight of the body is placed upon the lightly constructed atlas and cervical vertebrae rather than upon the heavy and massive lumbar vertebrae. This can be especially dangerous when the upper cervical bioductory sectors have been previously damaged and anatomically disordered.

Only the fit can survive a heavy course of body yoga as it is practiced by the masters in India.

Most chronically ill persons will profit from performing some limited physical exertion. Often, however, they prescribe for themselves a rigorous course to regain a slim figure and youthful buoyancy. Driving a weakened, chronically ill body to unnecessary and unusual amounts of physical exertion can lead only to increased trouble.

Pleneurethic is in no way opposed to physical culture, but true physical culture does not overtax the body. It does develop body symmetry, good posture, and body awareness.

Ordinary relaxation is easily achieved by anyone who has proper posture and who is not chronically ill.

All normal people automatically relax muscles not in use. Relaxation for those who have chronic bioductory damage is difficult, often impossible. Neural damage which leads to chronic illness also causes muscles (skeletal, visceral, and vascular) to be in a perpetual state of tension. The pattern of tension depends on the stresses in the central neural system.

With practice it is possible to direct consciously relaxing attention and specific awareness to the area of tension. As long as the attention is focused, the sensation of tightness and uneasiness with anxiety may diminish. However, when the attention is permitted to wander, the somatic tenseness returns, as does the chronic mental anxiety which accompanies it.

Directed conscious relaxation is useful but it is not to be confused with basic therapy—removal of the prime cause of chronic tension and the chronic illness accompanying it.

People do not habitually assume a slumping posture because they are lazy or indifferent. They may slump because their spine is unable to support itself in the proper posture, due to bioductory disorders from anatomical trauma, neural pathology, or because of osseous, ligamentous, and muscular changes. Such posture is often the result of an injury to nerve tract systems that disabled the skeletal branch of that nerve.

Modern overstuffed chairs are virtual torture devices. They are too large for proper sitting; too small for stretching out fully. The seats and back sags. They offer no proper anatomical support for the user. Many have a brace across the front of the seat that shuts off circulation of the blood in the lower limbs.

Chairs of proper dimensions are so constructed that the feet of the user touch the floor while the hips are touching the back of the chair. The seat and back are resilient but with good support. The back of the chair is angled for comfort.

An easy chair has arms of the correct height to absorb the weight of the user's arms, thus reducing the workload of the upper thoracic area.

Beds should be long enough to permit straightening the body to full length. They should also have support for the mattress that must not sag. Softness of the mattress is suited to the preference of the individual, but the mattress itself should rest on a firm foundation.

7

BRAIN-CULTURAL
RELATIONSHIP

So far we have been looking at Pleneurethic from the standpoint of the individual. Now we can move to a broader canvas and examine the possibility of destabilizing impact made upon people by cultures and human institutions and continue the discussion of Pleneurethic from the perspective of its social relevance.

Because Pleneurethic is concerned about the causes of mental and physical distress, it provides a platform for a study of stress-producing human institutions. It is possible for the collective neural systems of civilizations to be taxed by malstructured social institutions to the extent that widespread mental and physical disability may be produced when the unfortunate person brushes against them. In Pleneurethic these institutions must be looked at from the perspective of whether they contribute to a pathological departure from healthy reality and if so to what extent.

As already indicated there are many ways in which individual neural systems can be harmed. They can be affected by mechanical force accidentally applied to the body, and mauled by poisons or harmful drugs. They can also be menaced by excessive noise generated by jackhammers ripping into pavements, arising from busy airports, industrial plants, or city traffic. Neural systems are also jeopardized by poisonous pollutions coming from outside the body or generated within the body by chronic illness processes. Most assuredly they are imperiled by corrosive chemicals introduced into the body by the local brewery, or commercial pharmacy and its medical cohorts.

Man's neural system may also be adversely distorted by bad thinking, overwork, unremitting stimulation, insufficient rest, and other undesirable influences and situations. It can be further disturbed by some unrealistic religious doctrines, particularly as many persons who have intense but vague feelings of chronic neural irregularities feel that their god—whether he be the Christian or Muslim God, or Buddha—has deserted them. When they cannot ascertain a definite cause for their suffering they manage to convince themselves that they are being punished by a hostile god for some either real or imagined transgression. Unfortunately, such feelings are sometimes encouraged by religious advisers. But such fears are groundless although there are real, authentic, and demonstrable causes for such anxieties. These, however, arise from physical brain damage and not from some supernatural cause. Once the underlying reason for this uncertainty is pointed out to the sufferer and corrective action taken, the patient realizes that his fears of being forsaken by his God were groundless.

In Pleneurethic there is abundant faith in the divine. It is a faith based on the predictability and constancy of divine activity. Our faith is not based upon a wish that the divine will set aside some law or invoke a new one on our behalf, or that of our enemy. We do not believe that the divine issues special favors for us at the expense of others.

If we believe that the divine operates in mysterious and arbitrary ways we are lost. For mystery begins where prudence and understanding ends. The modern Christian church has been found by Pleneurethic to spawn much unconstructive worry and considerable harmful division of personal character. It is therefore indicted in those areas where it contributes more to the unhealthy splitting of the personality than to the integration of it.

It is also indicted for its high sophistication and deviation from absolute law, because this leads to loss of a realistic mental structure in the personality.

International Pleneurethic does not support any particular type of church or state. It contends that citizens must support their own state first, even though they are students of Pleneurethic. In this way Pleneurethic is definitely and unequivocally subordinate to the state. Whereas Pleneurethic itself is nonpolitical and nondenominational, people who subscribe to its tenets must abide by the laws of the country in which they live. To leave one's own state for the purpose of secretly subverting another is a scourge on earth and one of the gravest of all immoralities.

In Pleneurethic there are few freedoms or licenses but many responsibilities; no demands but many offerings; few rights or immunities, only duties; no special powers, only states of ethical being. Indeed, the greater our unilateral demand for unrestricted license, the more we are eventually restrained and restricted. Conversely, the more we assume personal discipline over our own self, the more expansive our ultimate freedom.

In Pleneurethic no race is inferior nor is any race superior. There is no criticism or hostility aimed at interracial marriages or their progeny. The poor are free to rise up if they ethically can without hindrance.

From this general discussion of Pleneurethic in the social context we can turn to an examination of some of the fields in which the adopted culture of modern society has thrown up problems which might be effectively approached through Pleneurethical mythodology.

Alcoholism: Pleneurethic offers substantial help to the alcoholic by showing where living stress is accumulating and why stress from one source reinforces others whose cause seems unrelated to it, to create an overall living problem of unmanageable proportions. Pleneurethic peels away the various layers of acute and chronic stress which combine to form the multilayered proclivity to alcoholism.

After the alcoholic recognizes his problem, and decides to take a serious step toward correcting it, he must face some facts. The first is that although alcohol does offer some temporary relief to a mind and body in distress, the effect is achieved by a toxic stunning of the neural system, more especially the brain. In the long term the neural system is harmed more by alcohol than the body and mind are helped. Indeed, alcohol adds its own layer of stress to an already overstressed neural system in the alcoholic person. Furthermore, excessive consumption of alcohol reduces our clear perception of reality because brain tissues are warped. Once our grasp on reality is distorted, our relationship with society may suffer.

Pleneurethical theory throws quite a lot of new light on predisposition to alcoholism. The new ideas are quite simple if we take the time to acquaint ourselves with some of the basic notions. The first of these is that the character, with its strengths, weaknesses, and predelictions, is influenced by the condition of the brain.

The second is that the brain is not an irrefrangible bulwark against all influence.

The third is the existence of the bioductory system, a flexible bony tube formed by holes through the vertebrae, which surrounds the neural system, to protect it. If this is chronically harmed, it imposes a direct mechanical strain on the central neural system which, added to other tensions of everyday life, creates havoc in body and mind. In such cases alcohol temporarily soothes the central neural system. The mind is pacified and the body relaxes a bit, but nothing of a permanent, curative nature has been achieved. Many unsuspecting people are encouraged to use alcohol by an accommodating media which lent itself to the glamorization of alcoholic consumption.

Addiction: Since the brain is the worldly window for the mind, we humans tend to get hooked and hung-up on things that assist or seem to assist brain performance.

When the brain is weak from the lack of proper nourishment, we like to eat. We also like to rest our brain when it is overtaxed, desensitize brain tissue when it registers pain or deep anxiety, and provide a source of stimulation when the brain is understimulated from boredom, or unproductive as a result of stupidity.

Sometimes the benefits from the source of stimulation we choose are more apparent than real. That which appears good at the time can have disastrous effects on the brain.

As illustrated earlier, the relief brought to the overtaxed brain by alcohol is achieved at the expense of the brain's sensitivity and the following morning brings a partial rebellion—headache and general nervousness. If alcohol is habitually consumed in large quantities the ensuing years bring premature decadence and death, and the process is even more rapid if neuralosis has already established a chronic deterioration.

Other drugs, such as LSD and marijuana, that enlarge the scope of the mind in one direction do so only by altering the microstructure of the brain and constricting the scope of the mind in many other directions.

Pleneurethic firmly opposes the use of any substance that artificially changes the scope of the mind, because it can do so only at the expense of the structure of the brain and our total mind.

To generalize, those people already debilitated from chronic illness may experience more disastrous consequences from small doses of toxin than healthy people. Normally dull people may tend to become addicted to agents which unnaturally excite brain tissue as people who are chronically hyperexcited may tend to become addicted to things which soothe their ailment. Besides alcohol and drugs, these panaceas can include overeating.

Although the brain furnishes the original grid upon which reality is displayed for interpretation by mind, mentality once structured also introduces its own bias to reality as this is interpreted by the mind. This is why the Pleneurethicist is interested in the structure of institutions as they affect the mind of man.

Motivation: In Pleneurethic we do not waste neural resources in an effort to show ourselves off to any particular advantage. Competence is rooted in our neural system. The fully competent, untraumatized brain interrelates easily with the mind. It does not reflect any instability or depression. It coordinates all our musculature both visceral and skeletal so that we are strong, well coordinated, and competent in all physical undertakings felt necessary or desirable.

We manifest our competence in a multitude of ways. We survive, but mere survival is not enough when the art of surviving becomes merely routine and is no longer a challenge. We demonstrate our competence by our power over others, our power over material, and our power over ourselves.

Fortunately, not everyone tries to evidence competence in the same way. Some develop themselves into good listeners, some into good talkers. Others play the piano, make money, catch fish, drive mechanical vehicles hard and fast, turn criminal —you name it. If two or more people try to show their competence along the same lines, competition results. This easily becomes constructive or destructive according to the rules of play and the line of the game. The Pleneurethical approach is the opposite of high competition and is a worthwhile goal of good ethical conduct.

Loss of Security: People feel a positive correlation between loss of security and their chances of survival. If one's living needs are being met, feelings of insecurity are not usually experienced, but when they do occur they are among life's most pressing problems. Loss of a job, children not loved by their parents, failure to pass examinations, enemy shells exploding in one's face—all such things of the real world and many more cause acute loss of security.

But there are some quite different causes. A person can feel very insecure most of the time, but cannot explain why. He or she may have no difficulty in meeting living needs, but will nevertheless feel chronically incomplete, unwanted, and uncared for.

One movie star had this form of loss of security. It was so severe that she consulted a psychotherapist for assistance. He gave her sleeping pills and tranquilizers to treat her physical symptoms and for her insecurity he prescribed building a strong home designed so as to give her a feeling of security in her life.

She built the home according to the psychotherapist's instructions, yet within a few months she was dead.

Actually, her loss of security could not be cured by changing her external environment, it came from inside her body and her chances of survival were slim indeed because the cause was not corrected. Her bioductory system was caving in on her neural system and destroying her somatic home; she knew the seriousness of her condition, but could not pinpoint the cause.

It is difficult to think of anything more horrifying than a condition wherein the bony casing around one's lower hind brain and life-giving spinal cord is slowly sliding out of control into insecure malposition. As the bony casing and the flexible bioductories crumpled, slid, slipped, corrugated, and turned rigid so as to destroy her neural system and the rest of her body and brain dependent on it, extreme loss of security was experienced. The personal terror that accompanies such a loss of security in one's life is difficult to document vividly. But it does exist and the terror is magnified by the incredulity, misunderstanding, and gross incompetence of orthodox physicians in the field of chronic illness and the attendant chronic anxiety.

The movie star did not receive Pleneurethic treatment and what would have been only a close scrape with death became an actual encounter, the grave digger being the only winner.

Frustration: Early training in encountering and handling general frustration is essential to producing well-balanced people. Frustration is an ever-present problem when people live together in a community.

Nowadays, frontiers have shifted from physical survival and achievement of comfortable living to something more nebulous. Children are no longer physically or economically frustrated as they were in the past. The dark forests have been cleared, the muddy paths paved, and the carnivorous wild beasts killed or beaten back. Children are given spending money for which they do not have to work. They are consulted on all matters and their opinions are automatically respected as though they had earned the right to speak out authoritatively.

The young are catered to far beyond the point that is good for them. The result is that when many of these young children become young adults and roll cosily out to overcome the outside world, they are ill-prepared to handle the occasional frustrations they meet. They do not see them as challenges that must be gracefully met and tactfully overcome. They do not see them as new forests to clear or new muddy paths to pave. Instead, they see them as the gross failure of the older generation who did not anticipate and clear away this last forest of despair. As a result they hate the older people and want to do away with them.

They call the sturdy policeman or college president—who is trying to do his job as best he humanly can—"pig." They are emotionally unhinged by any authority, especially the police, in this their first serious test of reality.

Pleneurethic advocates that criminality must be forestalled by early childhood training in the realities of life. Children should receive such training in the family, at school, and in the community. If they tangle with juvenile authority they should not be overprotected.

We must also recognize that some parents are at fault, not only in their failure to provide proper child training, but also in keeping themselves abreast of the modern movements.

No one is born a criminal, but children, if they are not properly trained in the realities of life, may overdemand. When demands are not met they often react in a temper tantrum and this pattern, if it is not checked, may be carried over into adulthood. Children must learn somewhere along the line that other people have rights. If they cannot achieve a grasp on reality the easy way, they must be taught the hard way.

Crime and Punishment: The Pleneurethical approach to understanding life's problems is rather complicated. If it were not complicated it would have been discovered and put down on paper years ago. What follows is the barest outline of my thinking on one of the most immediate problems of modern society. To understand my theory one must know something about how the mind works, a little bit about the brain and its neurological extension, as well as about the body and my discovery of the bioductory system and its ramifications.

With the key to understanding offered by Pleneurethic, the door to many puzzles of life can be unlocked.

It is a grave prejudgment to commence a study of crime by saying, "We will study the criminal mind." Frequently there is more in criminality than just mind. Mind is not an absolutely free entity able to change its basic course at will. It is largely dependent on brain tissue whose condition invariably exerts influence on the range and vigor of the mind.

To understand criminality we must appreciate that personality and character are more than a result of the mind, but include the influence of body and brain and early life experience as well.

There are also many classes of crime. The criminal may not have known that his act was unlawful. Here the correction is in the training of the potential criminal in the law of the land, simplification of statutes and uniformization of law within the various regions making up one state. The crime may have resulted from the overburdening of a normal person by complex living pressures that depress his brain capability for normal activity. The person then acts irrationally, injudiciously and perhaps criminally. A pressing situation demanding instantaneous evaluation and summary action may elicit a response which in the sober light of a courtroom becomes criminal in nature.

In a great many cases the capability of the person to withstand the pressing demands of modern living is diminished, not primarily by an unethical or criminal outlook or overburdening set of unusual circumstances, but by a chronic condition which causes the brain capability and mind performance level to be chronically depleted and unstable.

With certain patterns of bioductory disarrangement from, for example, accidents on the athletic field, the brain may be altered in such a way as to affect body biochemistry and the balance of hormones. The sufferer then becomes chronically ill and one of the symptoms could be abnormal feminization or masculization, with attendant sexual urges running contrary to the normal sexuality of the sufferer. Such people may manifest their nymphomania or homosexual tendency openly or they may keep it curbed, depending on their previous mental views on homosexuality. If they previously abhorred such conduct, afflicted people are often able to forestall making homosexual overtures or being receptive to such advances.

Pleneurethic can help the nymphomaniac or homosexual who

is not that way congenitally, nor because they want to try it for relief of boredom or kicks, but because a strange chronic malady has recently transformed or modified their body chemistry. But there are some abnormalities which, because they are congenital, are beyond the scope of Pleneurethic. The congenital idiot or moron may turn to criminal conduct because he knows no better, or the body, misshapen from birth, may goad the unfortunate person into various forms of criminality. The brain of the congenital idiot is structured in such a way as to produce permanent idiocy, as the body of the congenital monster is also formed from an ill-begotten mold.

Parenthetically, chronically ill parents who have been corrected Pleneurethically will create fewer congenitally defective offspring than those who have not.

In a very few instances of criminality, the brain is normally structured, the only congenital omission being a sense of ethic or a desire to get along well with other people. Such a person is again outside the scope of Pleneurethic because of his congenital ethical deficiency and congenital predeliction to trouble making and poor judgment in general.

Organized crime may come, not so much from chronic illness, as from leaders who are unethical. It is more an acute result of a malstructure of ethical mind than a chronic distortion or derangement of body. Here, the correction is to place each individual on his own responsibility for his own lawless conduct after he has been fully advised of the facts and consequences of his future decisions.

I am interested in promoting a society based on the economic use of a nation's collective neurological resources. The organized criminal is uneconomic because he could earn his living with less neural expenditure in the long run through honest ethical conduct than through dishonest unethical conduct. In the long run the hoodlum is consumed by worry, doubt, and fear, as are his potential victims.

Moreover, because of criminality, society must maintain vastly expensive penal and law enforcement institutions. There is a limit to the extent to which society can be drained to contain premeditated lawlessness. Criminality is neurologically uneconomic both for the individual bending his talent in that direction and for society which must now plan, erect, and maintain vast anticrime institutions to protect itself and to restructure the criminal mind when possible.

Neurological capability is our nation's most vital resource, and that which expends it uneconomically and unconstructively is a crime.

Education and training of prison inmates in a worthwhile trade is commendable, but many people seem to suffer chronic mental problems not because of lack of education, but because of chronic neural trouble and lack of neurological energy with which to power the declining and struggling mind. In this vital area of mind-brain relationship, Pleneurethic can be of inestimable value because it knows how to diagnose and treat mental problems no matter whether the cause is mental or physical. If a prisoner is chronically ill, it is more expedient to cure his chronic illness first and then teach him a trade than to train him in a trade and then turn him loose on society still acting atypically because of his uncured illness.

Pleneurethic does not recommend punishment for the sake of punishment. People guilty of real crimes should be corrected, not punished. However, the application of correction should be specific and heroic. A spartan atmosphere must prevail and a no-nonsense schedule of correction must be maintained. The ultimate correction, death, should be considered in cases where less drastic methods have failed and where the neural energy expenditures of society required for continued maintenance of the criminal far outweigh any prospective beneficial return from that particular person.

Life is not sacred. Life is a product of many factors but none of them are sacred. Inveterate hooligans and premeditated murderers and savage rapists who mutilate their victims are denied, in Pleneurethic, the argument that their lives are sacred. The world owes no one a living and no one may presume upon the good graces of the world forever.

Interrelationships between man and woman provide vast

areas in which malstructure of mind can occur, leading to acute anxiety in its most exquisite form. Much of such malstructure derives from impractical social custom, outmoded institutional marital regulations, and archaic divorce procedures. As our civilization moves forward through time and a changing technology imposes its profound influence on living patterns, basic rules concerning the relationship of men and women should also change, but in reality they have not changed sufficiently to meet new demands.

Pleneurethic sees a more realistic way of organizing fundamental relationships between men and women. This would recognize the needs of men and women as they actually exist in this modern era and would provide for further adaptation as times change. Marriage would be flexible, occurring in several different forms, and divorce would take different forms according to the type of marriage involved.

The first would range from occasional dates to casual living together and would occur because both persons enjoyed each other's company. The only thing agreed in this form of marriage would be the casual nature of the arrangement.

The second type would occur only after conception or birth and its purpose would be to establish responsibility for the support of offspring. Moreover, for each child there would be a new marriage covenant to establish responsibility, since different fathers might be involved in a succession of children from the same mother. There would be no divorce permitted in this second form of marriage since its only purpose would be to formalize parental responsibility; it would definitely not be a declaration of love or promise to support the wife herself as long as she might live.

If no father wished to marry a woman in her pregnancy, she could—if and only if she wished to—marry the state by signing herself into a Women's Corps. Here she would be subject to certain regulations with options as to the maintenance of the child after her release from the Corps. Duties in the Women's Corps would be commensurate with her ability and, if necessary, would include education and practical training for a future professional life.

The third form of marriage would be exclusively an ultrallectual union which could be consummated with no prescribed formal ceremony. No church or state can join people ultrallectually —they do it themselves as their sensitivities direct.

The fourth kind of marriage is purely a contractual business arrangement formalizing another relationship between man and woman which often arises from need through long association. It would include whatever contractual arrangements the two people concerned felt necessary. Divorce arrangements for the four types of marriage would vary according to the nature of the marriage.

The first could be broken off at any time by either party; the second could not be broken until the needs of the child terminated; the third, being perfectly flexible, is by its nature unbreakable; and the fourth could be ended or modified only through judicial proceedings.

The above cannot be construed as Pleneurethical law. It is simply the first faltering step in an attempt to create what could be a more realistic basis for meaningful interrelationships between women and men. As such it might help to reduce the incidence of stress, and improve chances for mental and physical health around the world.

Our earth's animal and plant kingdoms reflect and represent the basic array of forces in the universe and in turn are vulnerable to its vagaries as reflected, for example, in the changing seasons. This theme of structure and function is also manifested throughout the human species and it furnishes the prime basis for either health and well-being or chronic disorder and misery. More specifically, the structure of the human body and mind are correlated in Pleneurethic through the structure of the brain system. Each system influences the other and each distortion produces another to maintain biological equilibrium. However, there are definite limits to the proliferation of distortion that may be successfully entertained in any system. If this limit is exceeded for long, the life of the individual is lost through a process of collapse of the central neural system, leading to loss of that individual's structural abode on earth.

Defects of social, political, and economic institutions also reflect distortion to eventually induce stress in the individual and collective neural systems. It is for this reason that Pleneurethic is keenly aware of gross malstructure in such institutions. In the future, Pleneurethic may take an active role in the gradual reformation of institutions contributing to unproductive and unconstructive use of our civilization's neurological resources.

Pleneurethic is a bridge between East and West. Of course, the few hard-core Christians, the equally few hard-core Buddhists, as well as the remaining intransigents of the world religions, can never be expected to meet on common ground.

But there is great cooperative potential in the minds of the rational men of this world and such men are in the majority. Pleneurethic is an international avenue for common meeting, mutual understanding, and pure respect of all men of good will in all lands.

8

CASE HISTORIES
AND PREFATORY COMMENTS

PART 1

Pleneurethic postulates that chronic illness symptoms are mental interpretations of brain conditions and activities. *What sick people feel when they say they do not feel well is a mental awareness of the condition of their brain tissue.* If certain neurological tissues are upset, as they are in the chronic illness process, the mind feels or senses this cerebellar disorder and interprets it as not feeling well or being sick. These feelings are manifested by such symptoms as headache, nausea, dizziness, cranial heaviness, mental sluggishness, pessimism, and apprehension. They are definite neuromental mechanisms of the chronic illness process, a process not yet understood in pharmaceutical circles. Such feelings are definitely not mentoneurological machinations of some process imagined by orthodox medicine to be of an hysterical genesis evoked by an assumedly unsound mind.

Pleneurethic is perhaps more objective than any other healing science, but at first glance it may appear to be the least objective of all. For example, other healing sciences conclude that if the temperature and blood pressure are within limits, the patient has been cured. Pleneurethic makes no such assumption. Very often a patient with a normal range of temperature and blood pressure still complains of not being well and subsequently dies following severe exacerbations. Pleneurethic places substantial weight upon whether the patient feels himself to be sick or well and upon diagnostic findings of Pleneurethical significance concerning bioductory integrity and structure of the mind.

Other schools tend to consider the feeling of patients to be excessively subjective and unscientific. These schools have adopted this attitude out of necessity. They have never really understood the chronic illness process and therefore have erected their own systems of defense to counter certain therapeutic failures. In Pleneurethic no patient is sent packing with a bill for services rendered in one hand and a bottle of pain deadener and a stimulant or depressant in the other.

Feelings, which result from palpation of the brain by the mind, are regarded as natural by the person experiencing them. If the brain is chronically irritated and unstable, it is natural for the person to feel anxious, angry, and to be unsmiling most of the time. Just as it is natural, if the brain is placid and in good health, for the person to feel indefatigable and enthusiastic and happy most of the time. Much of the same is true of physiological activity. Depending upon the patterns of the brain's instability, it will seem natural to oversleep or undersleep, to overeat or undereat, or to be oversexed or undersexed. Just as it is natural for the healthy, stable brain to produce normal sleep rhythms and appetite for food and sexual feeling.

The point is that even though a chronically ill person does not particularly enjoy having a ravenous appetite or being a bit nauseated most of the time, there is little he can do about it. He will become obese or emaciated according to the eccentric drive of his chronically unstable brain. He will naturally eat all of the time or habitually decline food and there is nothing of curative significance that his mind alone can do about it. That which is true of the appetite for food holds true for the other biological functions. They all come under the influence of the brain. They act well when the brain is stable and perform unstably when the brain is ill.

Pleneurethic has been successful in reversing the cause of a number of chronic illness manifestations. In doing so, it has succeeded in partially relieving or totally eliminating a number of chronic illness complaints. Listed below are some of them:

* Chronic worry, fear, and loss of confidence replaced with feelings of well-being and optimism.

* Mental confusion replaced by the degree of mental clarity that existed before the onset of the complaint.
* Violent and persistent headaches replaced by a normal condition.
* An extreme loss of self-respect and lack of attention to personal appearance replaced with a normal level of self-esteem and attention to details of personal appearance.
* Numbness and paralysis eliminated from tissues of the face, ears, and neck.
* The number of colds suffered every year markedly reduced, and the severity of the colds which did occur were significantly reduced.
* Haggard and tense appearance of facial tissues replaced with a normal relaxed and more youthful appearance. Sagging or drawing of tissues on one side of the face corrected.
* Intense feelings of pressure inside the head or at the base of the skull abated and replaced by normal sensation.
* Nasal passages restored to normal caliber by reducing swelling of nasal membranes, and mouth breathing eliminated.
* Steadily deteriorating eyesight arrested and slowly returned to the normal condition which existed before the onset of chronic illness.
* Sudden, premature signs of age in facial tissues, progressing at an alarmingly rapid rate, retarded, arrested, reversed, and returned to normal condition for the person's actual chronological age.
* Severe muscular pain and stiffness in the neck replaced by normal mobility. Muscular weakness, joint pains, and loss of skin sensation in the hands or feet restored to normal.
* Fitful, nonrestful sleep restored to normal, restful slumber. Constant painful sensations in the abdominal areas eliminated. Tightness and constant feelings of apprehension in the chest area eliminated.
* Normal bowel action restored without the use of laxatives, special attention to diet, or use of abnormal amounts of nondigestible, slippery, nonabsorbable bulk fibers.

* Heavily engraved lines encircling the neck smoothed as cervical nerves and associated atrophied tissues returned to normal. Size of the neck increased as normal muscle tone and dimension was restored. Sagging skin on the neck tightened through the increased volume of cervical muscles and better tone of the skin.

PART 2

The physical signs that indicate that the bioductory system has been damaged vary considerably, depending on the location, severity, and length of time the damage has been consolidating and condition of visible tissues. Some of the early signs may be seen in mannerisms and affectations. Other signs are of a gross anatomical nature and are best ascertained by palpating with the fingers. Still other signs may be heard in the breathing, heartbeat, and speech.

Generally speaking, signs of bioductory damage can be divided into four types. These are:

* Physical signs presented by deranged anatomically injured areas in the bioductories.
* Neurological signs caused by bioductory-generated trauma in the central neural system.
* Physiological malfunctions and deteriorations in tissues and organs resulting from the central neurological trauma.
* Mental and behavioral characteristics stemming from chronic deterioration in the central neural system.

The bioductory system is susceptible to an infinite variety of traumatization patterns. The resulting pattern of damage to the brain is determined by the specific structural mechanics of the bioductory derangement. It is, therefore, difficult to list all of the points upon which bioductory diagnosis hinges—unless one is prepared to go into it in a professional way over a lengthy period of intensive study.

Basically, almost any chronic stiffness along the spine, neck, head, or hips denotes damage to some section of the bioductory system. Sometimes the sufferer only notices headache, a painful jaw that locks on occasion, pressure at the base of the head, yellowish or bloodshot eyes, or perhaps bursitis with subsequent arthritis in the fingers.

Sometimes nightmares, sleeplessness, fitful sleep schedules, or mental instabilities are indicative of chronic brain damage arising from bioductory system problems. Chronic anger or changes in perceptions of reality may also indicate bioductory damage.

As chronic bioductory trauma especially in the head, neck, and shoulder area causes chronic brain damage, chronic symptoms occur concurrently in the mind as mental illness and in the body as organic disorder. This explains why in such mysterious conditions as hysteria and psychosomatic illnesses, mental and physical illness go hand in hand.

Another sign to look for is the inability of the sufferer to be definite about his chronic complaint. This is because a person suffering from chronic brain malfunction and imminent tissue breakdown of a gross anatomical nature cannot be specific about the location of the source of his trouble. Moreover, he will be uniformly vague about the exact nature of his complaint and will change his story from day to day and year to year, especially in the early years of the history.

Further indications of bioductory trauma are: twisted posture, head cocked and held too far forward, tilted, twisted or too far to the right or left. One jaw that seems to be more prominent than the other gives a clue to suboccipital or cervical bioductory torsion. Heavy circular lines of tissue degeneration engraved in the skin of the neck, deeply engraved lines in the facial tissues, and chronic tension of neck muscles on one or both sides also point to bioductory damage, especially if they are noted early in life. Of course, all of these signs must be related to the person's age. They are more serious when they appear in young people. Chronic tics and sudden jerks of the head, neck, and body of an habitual nature are also signs of bioductory problems with attendant brain malfunction. Physiological signs run the full course of every conceivable form of chronic illness, from hypersexuality or perversion in the initial stages to final stages of impotency and frigidity. There may be immediate or delayed appearance of paralysis, mysterious rash, or chronic intestinal disorder.

Whenever a person experiences heavy physical trauma from an accidental fall, severe car whiplash, or is hurt by incompetently used obstetrics at birth, there is bound to be some degree of bioductory system damage. The portion of the bioductory system damaged and the extent of the damage depends upon the nature and severity of the injury.

Almost everyone at some time of his life has had an accident that could damage his bioductory system.

People who have ever been near children have at one time or another seen a child fall heavily from a horse, chair, or a tree, and been shocked when it lies still. They are relieved when the child cries and more so when it begins running around as if nothing had happened. The fall may have caused structural damage to the bioductory system which will change the whole course of its life. Shortly after such an accident a healthy child may be transformed into a sickly one suffering from a myriad of aches and pains and a general feeling of debility. The symptoms may be dismissed as some childhood growing pain and nothing to worry about. But as the child grows older the symptoms are likely to intensify.

Young men are often injured when they play violent sports and are sometimes knocked into temporary periods of unconsciousness. It is not unusual for them to suffer strange and chronic headaches, emotional disturbances, and general debilitating constitutional symptoms following a jarring experience on the sports ground. Damage can also be caused through falling on slippery surfaces and diving into shallow water. The aftermath of such accidents is often one of slow regression into a state of chronic ill health. On other occasions the bioductory disorder may be so severe that it will kill in a matter of days or weeks with the unfortunate victim passing through stages of high fever, convulsions, and sudden paralysis or coma. The lifting of very heavy objects when standing in an incorrect posture can also contribute to bioductory collapse which will damage cell bodies and tracts in the central neural system and spinal nerve roots and cause associated muscular or glandular organs to degenerate later in life.

The Pleneurethicist uses physical counterpressure to restructure bioductory disorders, but there is a tremendous philosophical and practical difference between his approach and orthodox recoil manipulative adjustment and massage treatment used by other healing schools. The Pleneurethical corrective counterpressure mobilizes and moves entire sections of the bioductory system into their proper position by the exertion of a measured, controlled, and properly vectored force which breaks down osseous adhesions, soft tissue strictures, and fibroses.

The recoil thrust adjustment, on the other hand, is a concussion of forces which aimlessly shakes and vibrates the spinal column. It is applied with the hope that the natural innate adaptive resources within the spine will be brought into play and the spine will adjust itself.

If the bioductory system is only acutely out of proper posture, readaptive forces will be built up along the system to pull it back into proper position. However, the natural intrinsic and inherent tendencies of the system to be normal are not omnicompetent and are never sufficiently adequate to correct chronic conditions without outside help. In chronic conditions the bioductory system loses its ability to respond fully to the normal readaptive forces which dwell in the neural establishment. The power of the innate adaptative forces deployed along the tissues of the system is also drastically reduced. Moreover, normal tissue mobility is lost to a chronically sick bioductory system. Needless to say, the patient, after a recoil adjustment, will be very stimulated and may mistakenly feel that something good has been done for him. However, after a series of stimulative adjustments have run their course, the patient may be little better if not worse off than before. Many people who practice general spinal manipulation find that additional therapeutic measures are required.

Pleneurethical correction, on the other hand, is invariably nonstimulatory. It is healing because it restores the capacity of the brain to carry out its structural and functional organization. To perform it is perhaps more difficult and exacting than knife surgery. The person doing it must possess exquisite judgment, a refined diagnostic ability, and consummate corrective skills. I do not intend in this volume to detail the curative methods employed by Pleneurethic as unskilled people may be tempted to try them out with what could be disastrous results. This is especially so because the procedures for correcting inner bioductory corrugations, fixations, shelvings, compressions, and disc protrusions appear simple in theory. Nevertheless, in practice they are inexpressibly difficult.

They require a type of forceful application designed to remove bioductory system malstructures deliberately and accurately. This Pleneurethical correction restructures the bioductory system and does not initially rely on the spine's innate adaptive forces to play a major role. But once the bioductory system has been redeployed, the innate metabolic forces are able to take over and complete the job, carrying away the debris which accumulated around the area when it adapted to the distortion which caused the original problem.

X rays are always useful as an assistance in determining a number of things about bioductory disorders.

Recent accidents may have created fractures in osseous tissues which have not yet healed. Fetal abnormalities may preclude proper formation in osseous tissues which form bioducts. It sometimes happens that the arches or lamina of vertebrae forming the bioducts have not properly formed. Under these conditions it may be better not to apply any heavy restructuring force, the same as it would be if there were any unhealed fractures present in the area. But because X ray can only cast a shadow and because it is dangerous in prolonged applications, X ray has a limited use in diagnosing bioductory damage and tracking the progress of therapy. The segments of the bioductory system are very complex arrangements and their exterior surfaces and articulating do not show up well on any single X-ray shot.

Masterful palpation and other skillful observations by a person of true doctoral capability are the only reliable ways to accurately diagnose bioductory system damage.

Early signs of bioductory system damage may be determined in detail by palpation, and generally by noting how the carriage of the body has departed from normal because of the accident. Later signs may still be determined by palpation, but arthritic consolidations, strictures, and hardening muscles may obscure the damage to all but the highly trained diagnostician. At this time many visual signs have developed on the external surface of the body. Such signs include areas or lines of tissue degeneration and exterior evidence of bone pathology.

To be really able to administer Pleneurethical treatment measures it is not only desirable but mandatory that the art of palpation be mastered. Palpation must be carried out before each use of restructuring force. It must also be used directly after the application of force to determine the effectiveness of the treatment. Palpation is necessary because one must know what to do and how much has already been done. There is no substitute for the highly developed skill of palpation. X rays can never replace it. However, before palpation can be mastered one must possess a consummate knowledge of the details of anatomical structures.

Moreover, since some Pleneurethical treatment involves restructuring the mind, the operator must understand psychic structure as well.

Recovery indicators (physical, mental, and behavioral) are the hallmark of Pleneurethic. These signs are of neurological and somatic regeneration and are usually first noticed subjectively by the individual himself and later by his friends. The person administering the Pleneurethic technique will also be aware of what is happening to the patient's neurological and bioductory system, but he will not be as conversant with the details of the behavioral changes.

There is a definite and distinct relationship between recovery indicators and the symptoms of chronic illness which previously marked periods of degenerative exacerbation. The recovery indicators are simply signs that the microstructure of the brain and function of a nerve tract that was once highly irritable, nearly inert, or imbalanced and certainly pathological, is being restored. These signs are evidence that the trend of structural and functional deterioration has been reversed and that a new era of biological reconstruction is commencing.

As the formerly pathological nerve cell bodies in the brain and nerve tracts regain their original vigor and normal neurological communication is restored to pathological somatic tissues, the person will notice that the organs relive or retrace the previous patterns of degeneration. Thus, old aches and pains and emotional disturbances which marked the original downward path of chronic illness will be experienced in reverse order. It seems that, as the person begins to climb back out of the black hole of chronic illness through the Pleneurethical restoration of his neural integrity, he must ascend the same path and reencounter in reverse order the same type of unpleasant experiences which previously marked his descent.

There are several redeeming features of this method. Not only is the person returning to a state of health, but the periods of discomfort are of a shorter duration and less severe than those originally experienced. The following case history of a middle-aged patient with a severe problem in the bioductory system affecting his brain and cervical and upper thoracic spinal cord nerve tracts will perhaps serve to illustrate this point. The man's history included a hand condition where the skin had been sensitive for years. This was followed by the loss of sensation in the skin of his hands. The joints of his fingers were enlarging and becoming quite painful. The strength of the muscles of the hand began to fade rapidly about the same time as the skin lost its feeling. Heavy ridges appeared on his fingernails, which became paper thin and curled to follow the contours of the tops of his fingers.

His case was a difficult one and about five months of treatment were required to achieve a definite and perceptible degree of bioductory structural improvement. On one particular day during the fifth month of Pleneurethical care a breakthrough was obtained in the lower cervical problem. On the following day the man reported that the skin and muscles of both his hands felt as if they had suddenly come alive and were being stung by a hive of bees. This most unpleasant but highly gratifying recovery indicator condition persisted for about forty-eight hours. Following this experience normal skin sensation, tone, and color began to return rapidly to his hands. The joints became progressively less painful as the muscles became stronger. The fingernails became strong, straight, and smoother. Indeed, before the breakthrough the muscles were so weak that he found it tiring to hold a knife and fork at mealtimes. Within eight months following the breakthrough the tissues of the hands were entirely normal. There was also a definite improvement in the condition of the skin on the back on the hands, which had been sagging and wrinkled.

The recovery indicators in this instance were the sensation of being stung by bees on the hands and an occasional very intense and massive pain in the muscles and joints of the hands which diminished as recovery progressed.

Recovery indicators may be noticed in any tissue of the body affected by chronic illness. They may be visible and objective or they may be entirely subjective and of a sensory nature only. For example, one patient had a persistently painful and uneasy feeling across his abdomen around the liver and spleen after a heavy attack of hepatitis. After being accepted for Pleneurethical care the uneasy condition seemed to subside over the months with therapy. However, on one occasion after nerve tracts and associated bioducts had been positively mobilized, he experienced heavy distress in the upper abdominal region. This lasted a few days and was followed by complete and permanent relief from his earlier symptoms. The recovery indicator in this case was the renewed feeling of abdominal distress for a short period directly subsequent to a marked increase in neurological communication from the brain to the hepatic tissues.

Some recovery indicators are quite dramatic and others are so unobtrusive that they pass wholly unnoticed. This is illustrated by the case of a man whose face and scalp were becoming progressively paralyzed. His condition was accompanied by terrible emotional problems. After some months of correction and after the paralysis was beginning to lift, the man noticed the sudden appearance of a painful and horny growth on the skin of his scalp. He paid no particular attention to it except to avoid it while combing his hair. After a few days he recollected that more than forty years before, when a young child in the early portion of grade school, he had been troubled with exactly the same type of growth in the same position on the scalp.

The recovery indicator in this case was the horny skin growth which reappeared within a few days after a particularly good advance was made in relieving traumatizing bioductory disorder on suboccipital and midcervical neurological tissues. Following this recovery indicator, the lifting of the paralysis was very rapid, as was the reestablishment of a more normal emotional tone, and skin tone of facial tissues.

People who have had dental extractions will often comment on recovery indicators which appear as heavy pain in the exact area of the jaw where the extractions were made years before. Such recovery indicators, when they appear, follow correction to brain-bioduct problems in the cervical region. Of course, it is too late to be of material assistance to a tooth already removed, but other teeth in various stages of degeneration may be assisted because the rate of future dental degeneration may be retarded. We rush to note that carious teeth even though properly filled may also become quite painful for a few days following a breakthrough in bioductory reconstruction. The gums may also be temporarily affected.

Readers having experienced dental operations will remember that each tooth has neural innervation which can produce real agony as the tooth is filled, extracted, or dies from a carious condition. These are the nerves which are affected by correction in the cervical area through a concatination of complicated biological events. There is a definite connection between nerve tracts in the cervical area and branches of nerve tracts which proceed from the brain to the gums and teeth. Parenthetically, the nerves to the gums and teeth also control their blood supply. The health of the teeth and surrounding tissues including the gums and jaw are easily caused to deteriorate through incomplete brain-nerve control due to anatomical structural disorder problems in certain areas of the bioductory system.

Recovery signs are always reversals of the symptoms of

various stages of the original chronic degenerative illness. The most important one being a knowledge that he or she is now getting well rather than knowing that he or she is unexplainably ill. Often the person has forgotten the various stages of pain and unpleasantness through which his organic establishment passed on its declivitous path into ever deeper manifestations of chronic illness. The reversal of the degenerative process, through the restoration of complete neurological fidelity to the affected regions, is often uncomfortable but it is necessary if a cure is to be achieved. One must expect difficult periods during the course of Pleneurethical care. It is only fair to list them at the outset.

There may be brief local pain at the time restructuring force is applied. No anesthetic is used during a Pleneurethical correction and the pain, if it occurs, will be at the exact point to which the force is administered. The pain lasts only for a split second when it occurs and then vanishes. But local stiffness and some tissue soreness may manifest itself for a few days following the initial treatments. Some persons develop strange sensations, aches and pains perhaps in remote regions, which may persist for a few days or weeks. These pains are not always at the point where restructuring force was applied, but are, nevertheless, a result of the force. The pains may be moderately severe and can be even frightening.

If the individual tries, he can usually recall the back pain which accompanied the accident which disorganized the section of the bioductory in question. To avoid the pain and to stabilize the malpostured area, nature commenced to immobilize the damaged area of the bioductory system. The bioductory system remained immobile in a disordered structural position, but relatively painless through loss of normal neurological communication until Pleneurethical procedures began to reverse the process. Before Pleneurethic can reestablish the normal position of a partially malpositioned section of the bioductory system, it must be mobilized and shifted into orderly relation with other bioducts. This process may introduce severe to light pain lasting for a few days to a few weeks.

During the first weeks or months of Pleneurethical care, immobilized bioductory tissues may remain motionless and painless. However, once the bioductory tissues begin to move under Pleneurethical management, there may be considerable pain connected with each movement. There will be pain as the force of correction is applied, and there will be pain as the individual moves these tissues during normal living body movements.

When this type of pain appears, the individual should not overly favor the painful area of the bioductory system because it is now in an anatomical position to profit from normal or near normal exertions based on the rate of progress of regeneration. If the painful bioductories, after receiving treatment, are inordinately favored, the time required for successful completion of the case will be prolonged. The thing to remember is that it is normal and natural for the tissues adjacent to an immobilized area of the bioductory system to become painful for a period of time as mobility and neural communication begins to reappear.

Tissues surrounding a normal section of the bioductory system are painless if Pleneurethical pressures are exerted upon them. They have normal response and if they are occasionally given Pleneurethical attention there will be absolutely no pain as the bioducts are moved.

On some occasions a very serious bioductory injury will result in total loss of sensation with great loss of tissue tone in associated tissue areas. Even when such areas are mobilized Pleneurethically there will be absolutely no pain whatsoever until, following some period of delay, nerve endings in adjacent tissues commence to regenerate. In a way, these types of injuries are more serious than those immediately painful following initial correction.

Pain from the force of treatment at the time of application is variable, depending upon the state of tissues involved and the temperament of the person. Many people do not feel pain at any time. Others feel pain but comment to the contrary. Still others will magnify the slightest pain when discussing it with acquaintances, their temperament being to howl and scream at the least discomfort. If pain does accompany the treatment force, it is of an instantaneous nature, completed in a fraction of a second.

Thus, there are two possibilities of pain associated with the Pleneurethical treatment: the instantaneous pain of a very short duration, appearing at the time force is applied; and the second type of pain, which is a relatively long-lasting condition associated with somatic tissue recovery from chronic illness. This second type of pain may be noticed over a period of several weeks each time the body is flexed in the area that is undergoing repair. When pain does appear, it can come in any month during the course of Pleneurethical care when the restructuring breakthrough is achieved. Persons experiencing pain should comment on its presence and where it is felt the most especially, if severe. It may become necessary to suspend work on one particular area of the bioductory system for a time while it goes through stages of regeneration after mobilization or partial mobilization. However, time is not lost in this event because there are usually other areas which can be profitably worked on, and tissue regeneration proceeds at its own pace once neurological fidelity is restored.

The trend of improvement in health and well-being is not a smooth upward path. There will be reverses. There will be days when the individual will feel that no progress with his case has been made and he may actually feel in a worse condition than before. On these days there will be brief but intense periods of disappointment and discouragement. The course of Pleneurethical care is quite lengthy for some seriously ill persons. People who are in very advanced stages of chronic illness may take several years to cure. No one can really expect to keep only a few appointments for a week or two and leap to a sudden and complete recovery, although this does happen on occasion. But cases are not accepted on this basis. The road to real and permanent health can be long and trying, but it can be negotiated with Pleneurethic.

When brain integrity is restored Pleneurethically, organic structure and functions which were previously depressed by the chronic cerebellar degeneration do not improve uneventfully. Considerable time is required for the damaged neural system to rebuild its capability and reestablish its normal biological stability on a full and complete level of competency. There will be periods of overcompensation followed by short intervals of undercompensation as the brain seeks to establish normal equilibrium both within itself and the peripheral somatic tissues which it governs.

As neural response and brain energy sufficiency are improved and stabilized on a higher level of efficiency, somatic and psychic changes will also occur. These functional changes will make wide, seemingly uncontrolled, gyrations from overactivity to under-activity as progress toward total recovery is achieved. The amplitude of these temporary and seemingly erratic overcorrections and undercorrections will gradually diminish as will their time duration. For example, chronic constipation may be replaced by brief periods of diarrhea before normal bowel actions are established. Chronic sleeplessness may be replaced by brief periods when the person may sleep all night and most of each day for a time before a normal sleep rhythm is restored. Skin areas of the body which may have become insensitive and numb may feel as if they were covered with a hive of stinging bees before normalcy is restored. Ribs which have been inactive and without sensation for years may pass through periods characterized by heavy rib pains when pressure is placed on them in lifting, coughing, or just standing straighter. Persons who have become docile and sub-missive due to their illness may pass through a temporary period when they project considerable aggressiveness, hostility, and perhaps even domineering forthrightness.

There will be other intense, but short-lived, reversals of previously abnormal symptoms as the vital capacity of the neural system cycles the functioning physiology of the body through a series of underadaptations and overadaptations whose amplitude becomes successively less until the normal stability of the neural and related tissues is well established. Structural improvements of tissues and organs occur.

Pain and other generally unpleasant sensations are experienced when organic tissues in previously unnoticed areas of the body are stretched, expanded, and strengthened by structural regeneration as the neurological communicative influence is restored to normal. As the nerve tissues of the spinal cord in the cervical area are relieved of chronic bioductory disorder there may be a short period which is characterized by a sore throat and nasal discharge. But organic operations which were unaffected by the chronic illness will also be unaffected by Pleneurethic treatment and will not register any of the recovery symptoms.

Not all of the unpleasant rejuvenative indicators are experienced by every patient. Many patients feel no discomfort whatsoever. They simply begin to regain a feeling of optimistic well-being. Moreover, there are many pleasant rejuvenative indicators such as increased energy, clear-headedness, increased libidinous energy, and optimism. The eyes become very clear.

One of the most pleasant and gratifying recovery indicators of an objective nature has to do with the appearance of the face. A renewed look of freshness usually accompanies Pleneurethical care. It can be stated, almost without exception, that each elderly, middle-aged, or chronically ill young person receiving Pleneurethical management has experienced at least a partial rejuvenation of facial skin and underlying muscular tissues. The most frequent comment that friends and acquaintances make to individuals who have been making Pleneurethical appointments is that they look years younger.

The reason for this de-aging process is that as the brain and nerves innervating the facial tissues become healthier and stronger, they encourage an increased flow of blood to the facial tissues. This in turn restores voluptuousness and tonicity to the facial muscles. The tone of the facial skin is also improved and its general health is increased. As the facial skin become more elastic it draws tighter over the now healthier and more rounded facial muscles. Wrinkles disappear, and the skin loses its thin and parchment-paper-like appearance. It is better than a face-lifting operation because not only is the skin reinvigorated but the underlying facial muscles become less tense or flabby.

All chronically ill people who receive Pleneurethical care experience a subtle and important personality change. I have called it the "Self-Appraisal Shift." It is especially evident in persons who are relieved of suboccipital, cervical, or upper thoracic bioductory disorder. Persons suffering from long-standing chronic illness tend to lose their self-confidence and self-respect. After a period of time they feel they are less capable and valuable than they once were. With these devalued opinions of themselves they are willing to settle for less of the good things which life has to offer. They will often work for less money, take abuse from others, or accept the love of an inferior or unsuitable person. As their health is restored through the application of Pleneurethical measures the person will again reach a level where his opinion of himself becomes normal. Before reaching this level of self-appraisal, however, the person who previously placed an excessively low value on his capability and value may pass through a stage of rapid improvement, causing him to overestimate his value, ability, and worth. Thus, there may be a period when the person is overconfident and bestows excess self-esteem upon himself.

During the period marked by personality upgrading, the personality may alternate excessively as the regenerating brain and peripheral neural system endeavors to stabilize itself. The person will most probably have ups and downs of over- and under-self-evaluation and confidence. It is especially important that the person concerned should execute no decisive and important plans concerning himself, his business, or his loved ones during this regenerative period. This time is required for the previously degenerating neural system to reverse its trend and readjust and stabilize itself on new levels of health and balance. The personality shift period marks a chronic illness reversal and represents a changing era in the individual's life. Utmost care must be exercised in formulating and executing policies during these periods.

All chronic sufferers require sympathy from friends and the people they love. Frequently they receive the opposite because no external nor internal medical reason for the sufferer to be ill can be seen. In fact, his or her friends may even feel that he or she is wallowing in self-pity, and is trying to elicit their sympathy. They may judge the sufferer to be hysterical, deceitful, malingering, or to be an excessively weak-charactered person who just needs to "buck up" and face life resolutely, optimistically, and confidently. Such friends, unfortunately, will merely intensify the suffering of the stricken individual. This attitude arises mainly because people do not usually realize that illness can be divided into two general types. The first is an acute type which results from accidents and produces visible injuries such as broken bones, crushed organs, or gashed flesh. From this type of illness the sufferer will receive abundant sympathy and support from his family and friends because there is substantial observable evidence to support his complaint.

The second type of illness is of a chronic nature, which manifests itself in a subjective sort of way in the beginning. Although the person suffers from a legitimate, if misunderstood pathology, there is no observable reason for him to be ill. There is nothing patently evident for people to recognize as a valid reason for illness. Hence, other people are uniformly unresponsive with constructive advice, helpful assistance, or sympathetic understanding. Family and friends of the sufferer lose their patience as the illness drags on through the years, with its characteristic periods of exacerbations and remissions. To make matters worse, doctors usually say there is no medical reason for the person to be ill. There is little wonder, then, that the sick person should feel rejected, misunderstood, unneeded, and even unwanted.

As the person becomes increasingly ill from, say, a chronic suboccipital or cervical bioductory disorder and the brain deterioration which attends it there are pronounced personality changes. But by the time these occur associates and others may be reacting with hostility and sarcastic advice rather than supplying much needed understanding and assistance. Such inattention intensifies the chronically ill person's suffering and perhaps accentuates his resentment. Under such tragic and heartbreaking circumstances he is likely to consider such terrible things as suicide or else will demand exploratory surgery in an effort to convince others that he is really ill. He needs respect and support, not hostility and ill-concealed contempt.

But such people can be helped by Pleneurethical corrective measures. It is essential, nevertheless, that the family and friends of people who suffer from chronic illness understand what is happening to the person and sympathize with him and help him. It is also essential that they understand the reversal effect that Pleneurethical care has on chronic illness.

Most persons under Pleneurethical care derive a great deal of satisfaction relating their experience with recovery indicators to other persons. Once properly understood, the recovery indicator is a sign of great importance to both the patient and those responsible for his care. Indeed, it is most beneficial to discuss recovery signs with others who are also under Pleneurethical management. By comparing notes, each person receives a greater insight into the wonderful things that are happening to the body, brain, and mind.

Perhaps the most significant recovery indicator of all occurs in the person's mind. The person intuitively senses that, instead of being sick, he can now be well. It is almost as if the person under treatment has at last generated the will to be well on his or her own. With this newfound premonition or subliminal urge, patients often feel that they can be healthy simply by willing it to be so and acting as if it were the case. Further outside help is neither required nor desired by the person once this spontaneous and irrepressible recovery process is experienced.

PART 3

The remainder of this chapter will be devoted to the discussion of individual cases. The first case was an actual incident although it was not observed at first hand by the author.

Case Number One

Mary was just twenty-one. She was of normal weight but seemed to lack energy although she ate well. She frequently complained about not feeling well but was unable to explain very clearly why. All she could say was that she felt very peculiar at times. She was examined by many doctors and was even committed a few times to psychiatric institutions for treatment. But the verdict from doctors and psychiatrists was always the same. There was nothing to worry about because tests showed her to be organically normal.

One evening at home she became unusually upset. Her family took little notice of her on this occasion because they knew Mary was a highly imaginative young girl with strange and groundless delusions of illness. After a late dinner, Mary told her mother she was sick. Her mother said she wasn't and told her to go to bed. Mary went to her room but returned shortly afterwards and asked her mother to press a painful spot at the base of the neck high up between her shoulder blades. The mother refused and told her daughter somewhat sharply to get to bed. She softened it by adding that she would take her shopping the following morning. Next day, however, Mary did not come down to breakfast. The mother went up to get her. She found her daughter dead in bed.

The death, following a routine postmortem examination, was attributed to heart failure. The pain in Mary's back and her reaction to it is interesting to us. The heart as well as other vital organs including pulmonary and cerebellar tissues receive neurological communication from nerve tracts. These transit the suboccipital and cervical bioducts and emerge from the spinal cord through lateral foramina in the bioductory system high up between the shoulder blades. During the last precious hours of her life Mary knew instinctively, in a hazy and general sort of way, what could be done to preserve her existence. Her death could have been from brain failure rather than heart attack.

Case Number Two

Jimmy was old enough to ride a bicycle. But he wasn't interested enough to do so. He was afflicted with one cold after another and had no energy. He spent most of his time inside the house reading and lying around while other boys around his age were outside playing. He took vitamins and other medicines, prescribed to stimulate him, regularly. Because his mother and father were well-to-do he was given the best of everything. His diet was perfect. It included a well-balanced supply of fresh, wholesome food. He ate little. He was thin but not emaciated. Even so, all his ribs could be seen in clear outline. He went to bed early every night but for some reason did not wake up refreshed with a boyish enthusiasm for life. He did not want to play any sport or take any physical exercise. He smiled wanly. He never shouted with mirth at some childish joke. He was serious but not quite grim or sedate. His family was starting to think he was a little bit strange but decided a good talking to was what he needed to give him a little starch like other boys. They knew there was nothing wrong with the lad as he had been examined by several doctors who had carried out several tests. These had shown no abnormalities.

Jimmy was brought for Pleneurethical care by his aunt. An examination showed that his spinal cord nerve tracts were damaged in the suboccipital and upper thoracic bioductory regions. The damage was caused by a traumatized bioductory structural disorder. Restructuring procedures were inaugurated to anatomically restructure the offending section of the bioductory system. Jimmy's responses were gratifying but not unusual. He seemed to blossom out over the weeks of therapy. His eyes became very bright and clear. He changed from a quiet retiring boy into one of the noisiest in his group. He began to run and play in a manner no doubt calculated to catch up on all he had lost. He rode his bicycle from morning to night. Muscles developed where nothing but skin and bone had been before. Two years after therapy, Jimmy had not had one cold nor could be found lying around reading or watching others play. He was too busy with his own boisterous games.

One of the interesting facets of Jimmy's case is that his parents, to this day, do not believe that Pleneurethic had anything to do with the transformation. They attribute the change in their son to the fact that he mysteriously but very naturally outgrew his previously shy and retiring ways. They know that his aunt took him to some sort of doctor whom they had never heard of before. But they consider his present healthy condition to be an outgrowth of the gradual disappearance of his sickly childlike shyness, which was naturally replaced by boylike boldness. In their minds it was time for this sort of change to take place in the boy's personality. It just took their boy a little longer to get going, but he finally did it all on his own. The parents are perfectly proper in their belief. Pleneurethic did nothing other than physically reverse the anatomical structural problems which were responsible for his improperly operating and pathological brain. Jimmy did the rest through the impetuous intensity of his physical play.

Case Number Three

Carol was the widowed wife of a successful real estate and oil man. She had two lovely children and was attractive at thirty-five. She was of medium height and moderately active. Over the past five years her desire for alcohol and narcotics had increased. She was frequently found in an incoherent state mumbling that she had to "break out." But she could not say what she wanted to "break out" from.

She was brought by a friend for a Pleneurethic examination. It disclosed severe nerve tract damage in the spinal cord at the base of the skull and midcervical region. Her condition was so serious that the skin on the back of her head just where it joined the upper neck would break down periodically into open sores. Her entire cervical bioductory area was extremely painful to the touch and she would not move her neck or turn her head if it could be avoided. She had been examined by many regular and irregular doctors. They noted nothing much out of the way that could be cured. Carol was taking tablets to strengthen her heart action, drinking intoxicants to stabilize her emotions, and taking drugs to derive some small satisfaction from her shattered life.

Carol elected not to receive Pleneurethical care because her neck was too painful. She decided that since she now knew the source of her trouble it could be best treated by massage and hot towels.

But in less than one year her death notice appeared in a local newspaper.

Case Number Four

The man was about fifty years old. He was a penniless laborer and he was brought by friends to test the effectiveness of Pleneurethic. When the man was in his late teens, he was taken to hospital suffering from a sudden and mysterious illness. The hospital had given no name to the disease but by the time he was discharged he had lost control of his voice.

He could now only grunt in a horrible way and saliva rolled out of his lips from the effort. His grunting could just barely be interpreted as words by his few close friends. Even so, he could not communicate at a rate greater than one or two words a minute. People avoided him. They did not want to be subjected to the tension build-up from his heartbreaking efforts to speak, or watch the terrible grimaces of his facial and neck muscles that went with the effort. The man had been in this condition for more than thirty years before he was brought to me.

A Pleneurethical examination revealed extensive problems in the upper cervical spinal cord nerve tracts and their associated major and lesser bioductories. I gave him treatment the first day at two-hour intervals. The following day I gave him three therapies. He received care on a daily basis after that. On the fifth day the man was positively beaming. His face was fresh and a jubilant smile was fixed on it. His acquaintances estimated that 75 percent of his speech had been restored. He commented that he could speak with less effort. Treatment continued until the disorder was reversed. Most cases do not respond as rapidly as this. It is not unusual for correctional procedures to be administered for one or two years. The length of time normally required to reverse a bioductory disorder depends on the age of the patient, the nature and location of the disorder, and how long it has been in existence.

Case Number Five

This is a very average case. In fact, it is an example of one of the most routine types of illness which are treated by Pleneurethic.

Jane was about thirty-five years old, a mother with one child. She had an excessive appetite and was physically plump. She suffered from severe headaches and was very dull witted. She had little initiative and could not work at any occupation requiring even a normal degree of mental activity and alertness. Her expression was listless and apathetic. She never laughed or smiled. She wore no makeup and her hair was always somewhat disheveled. She was brought for Pleneurethical examination. It revealed a moderate problem in the upper thoracic and cervical bioductory region. She was given Pleneurethical treatment every day for one week, then three times a week over a two-month period. After this, visits were reduced to twice a week for several months, then to once a week, and finally to once a month before the treatments were discontinued.

After the second week of treatment Jane reported that she had one day which was almost completely headache-free. After this she suffered a three-day bout of headache. But this attack was followed by two days of complete relief from it. This alternation continued until the headaches left her for good about one month after she began receiving Pleneurethical corrective treatment. She began to brighten mentally. Her eyes became clearer and her muddy complexion fresher. Within a few months she was getting her hair set at the neighborhood beauty shop. She also began to wear makeup. Her entire personality underwent a tremendous change. She became a laughing, vivacious woman in the prime of life. She was given a position of responsibility as a cashier in a large office and was promoted within a few months to a position carrying greater responsibility.

The only treatment Jane received was to the physical structure of major spinal cord bioductories in the upper thoracic and cervical regions.

Very little emphasis was placed on getting her to revise her life guidelines on a philosophical or psychological level because her intellect was quite normally structured.

The resurrection of Jane's personality was entirely due to her own initiative once her damaged brain and spinal nerve tracts were normalized. She received no pep talks, no special diet, no vitamins, no senseless forward-bending exercises, nothing but the restoration of the damaged malpostured bioductory system in the suboccipital and midcervical regions.

Case Number Six

According to her parents and friends, Joan had been a strikingly lovely girl in her late teens. At high school she had been an outstanding student excelling in mathematics, chemistry, and physics. Yet when I first met her she was about to be permanently committed to an institution for the insane. Her parents were preparing to sign the committal papers. She had already been before the medical board and her mental condition was judged to be beyond treatment and to be degenerating at a very rapid rate.

When she was brought to me her hair was unclean, uncombed, and dangling. Her eyes had a wild stare about them. A thick nasal discharge had nearly traversed the distance between each nostril and the upper edge of her lip. Her head bobbed forward in an impulsive movement, bringing her chin to touch her chest, and would then bob back into its normal position. It would do this every few minutes. Joan could speak, but in a fast, rushing manner which bordered on incoherence. She knew she was ill but was powerless to prevent the unrelenting and accelerating progress of her deteriorating condition. She was terrified by the steady decay of her faculties. She seemed to be able to sense the inevitable outcome of her condition if it were allowed to continue unchecked. She had a ravenous appetite and suffered from headaches. She also found it difficult to sleep. She thought she slept less than two hours every night.

Her friends had long since deserted her. She was anxious, fearful, and had lost every vestige of self-confidence. She clung desperately to any small thing which would brighten her miserable day. She tried to befriend everyone and anyone. But no one was interested.

I inaugurated measures to restore a severe anatomical structural disorder of the bioductories that was affecting the brain and spinal cord tracts in the cervical and upper thoracic area. In the beginning nothing much happened but after three weeks of treatment Joan suddenly became relaxed and sleepy. She did nothing but sleep on and off for two weeks. She slept all night and napped often during the day. So intense was her requirement for sleep that she became alarmed that she might sleep her life away and be worse off than before.

In a few more days her sleep rhythm became more normal; as it did, so Joan began to notice her appearance. She started to change her clothes before too many food spots collected on them. One day she tried a little lipstick. The next day she combed her hair slightly. From then on she began to pay a little more attention to her appearance each day. By the end of three months she was a model of young female beauty. Her hair was neatly arranged and her makeup expertly applied. Her confidence was restored and she reported that she had begun to resist the degrading orders issued by her mother and older sister. These orders had at one time perhaps been necessary, but they had gotten out of hand during the horrible days of her terrible illness. As a result of the change in her, Joan's parents never got around to signing the committal papers.

The last time I saw Joan she announced she was going to graduate from a medical school. I am sure she will make a very enlightened and competent doctor. She knows without question what it was that restored her to the world of the living.

Case Number Seven

This is another case where chronic brain illness affected the mental and physical condition. I am including it to show the different patterns such diseases can take.

When Jackie was brought to me she sat perfectly rigid, staring fixedly straight ahead. She seldom spoke. When she did it was in a crying, high-pitched, hysterically intense voice. She understood what was said to her and her answers were logical. She said most of her time was devoted to thinking through the numbers from one to four in endless repetition.

Her family and friends tried to help her by telling her time and time again to stop sitting still and to go out and meet people and enjoy herself like other young women. They kept reminding her that doctors, who had seen her, had said there was nothing wrong with her and her whole attitude sprang from an overfertile imagination. In other instances they accused her of being lazy and finally told her that she was just acting stiff and funny because she wanted to do so.

I found Jackie to be a thoroughly frightened and dismayed young woman. She knew she was trapped by some unnatural enemy that was forcing her rapidly into a darker, deeper inescapable corner. She fully realized that in her worsening condition she was of no use to herself, her children, or her husband. Her chronic anxiety and fear, which at one time had been modified by hope and faith, had long since given way to chronic anxiety and fear modified by utter despair. Only her fine character prevented any display of resentment or anger from her.

It was a wonder that Jackie, knowing the extent of her illness, did not become violent when her friends told her she was not sick and that all she needed to do to get well was to rearrange her crazy thinking in an orderly way like the rest of them. Instead of getting violent, Jackie sat it out for a while.

The night before the day of Jackie's first appointment for Pleneurethical examination she took forty sleeping pills before going to sleep. She was rushed to hospital for emergency pumping of her stomach contents. She remained in hospital for six weeks and immediately she was discharged was brought to me for a Pleneurethical examination. The examination revealed a massive disorder in the middle cervical and suboccipital section of the central neural system. This condition arose from bioducts that were traumatically malstructured. As a result direct physical pressure was being pathologically exerted on the lower border of the base of the hind brain and the upper reach of the spinal cord, and the flow of blood to the brain was also being interfered with.

Pleneurethical measures were instituted immediately to the pathological suboccipital and middle cervical bioductory area.

Jackie was also assisted and supported by being complimented in front of her family for her courage and strength in meeting such a horrible illness in such a commendable way. She and her family were informed that counting from one to four was a very practical way to use her mind in a case of such extreme physical and mental illness as hers. I told Jackie she had nothing to be ashamed of. If any other members of her family had been similarly afflicted they may have acted in a much worse manner than she had.

She was strengthened by knowing that someone had actually found something wrong with her, and was doing something to fix it. The knowledge raised her own self-esteem. She no longer had to face the patronization of her friends. On their part, once her friends realized that she did have an actual physical problem, they hastened to give her sympathy instead of thoughtless and unintended abuse. In three months of treatment Jackie made remarkable progress and is now nearly as well as she had been years earlier when she started to become ill and withdrawn and rigid.

The recovery indicators which she registered during the third week of her treatment were especially interesting. She suddenly snapped out of the extreme state of rigid lethargy and became very excited and jittery. She could not calm herself down long enough to receive corrective treatment. This condition lasted for two days. Then normal treatment schedules were resumed.

No effort was made to correct Jackie's thought patterns,

goals, and evaluation standards through verbal therapy for they were basically normal. Her only real abnormality was the pathological condition of the cervical bioductory system, spinal cord and distal end of the medulla oblongata. The other abnormality which existed in her environment was the understandable but absurd and injurious analysis placed on her condition by friends and professional healers.

Case Number Eight

Katherine complained of sleeplessness, headaches, and a painful heart condition for which she took drugs. Her eyesight, which had been normal during childhood, now caused her difficulty. She was twenty-five years old. Her most vexing complaint was her extreme anger, which turned into rage despite her desire to control it.

Katherine was a walking volcano which belied her exquisite face with its look of innocence. She was angry all of the time. She managed to keep it subdued as best she could but at the slightest provocation she would lose control. Her friends knew her to be dangerous and were careful not to antagonize her in the slightest way.

She realized her problem and of her own volition spent several months in a quiet refuge seeking help. Here she attempted to develop the willpower to suppress her rage as well as to adopt a peaceful, inner philosophical calm. However, after leaving the institution she again noticed that the slightest provocation would engender a temper outburst that was evidenced by instantaneous and uncontrollable rage. Katherine's eyesight seemed to be degenerating in inverse proportion with a corresponding increase in her propensity to rage and sleeplessness.

A Pleneurethical examination showed that Katherine had several different areas of bioductory system damage and pathology affecting the tissues of the central neural system. The upper cervical, upper thoracic, lower thoracic, and lumbar spinal cord areas were all affected. The brain itself was also being pathologically influenced.

I accepted her case for treatment and commenced procedures

immediately. The treatments were extended over a period lasting close to a year. Excellent and gratifying results were obtained. Some of them were astonishing and had not been predicted. As expected, her eyesight improved, as did the sleeeplessness and frequent headaches. The constant state of anger and rage also cleared away after one spectacular and venomous outburst which lasted three days. Her emotions then became normal and placid. She was not easily aroused to anger. If she did become angry she held it in abeyance easily and it was always a normal reaction to a provocation which would have aroused a similar response in any healthy person.

Toward the end of the course of her visits, Katherine said she had stopped taking her heart tablets and that painful lumps in her breasts had disappeared. These lumps had been bothering her but she had not complained about them in her original visit. Katherine had also kept secret one additional symptom of a more personal nature. She reported that she was no longer as desperately interested in men as she had been. According to her, her sexual appetite had been insatiable. However, over the past few months she had been able to control her erotic passions and was now able to permit them freedom only when it served her premeditated purpose.

It would almost appear that Katherine's rage was similar to sham rage, which can be demonstrated clinically in animals by severing the fibers which connect the cerebral cortex and the hypothalamus. Katherine had in effect been biologically de-corticated by pathological complications arising from nerve tract damage in her spinal cord. During treatment nerve fibers from the upper thoracic sympathetic outflow which ascend through the inferior, middle, and superior cervical ganglion and pass back inside the skull in company with the intervertebral and internal carotid arteries, had engineered the regeneration of great and important areas of brain tissue. As a result her hypothalamus had been rejuvenated, along with the cerebral cortex and interconnecting nerve tracts. The neurological mecha-nism of the eye, including the optic nerve, was also regenerated. The process also affected the optic tract and chiasma which are connected to the visual interpretation centers in the occipital lobe of the cerebrum through the lateral geniculate body and optic radiation. As a result her eyesight improved.

In time the neural tissues, blood vessels, and supporting tissues in Katherine's brain were restored to their normal biological structure and function. There is a tremendous amount of anatomy and physiology connected with eyesight and in Katherine's case it had all improved. As the function of her neurological tissues improved the mechanism of rage abated.

Case Number Nine

Frank had been a boxer in his youth and had even done a little professional fighting. He was now, at forty-five, a successful businessman. But he had trouble with his breathing. He would have an asthma attack at intervals of perhaps a week. No matter which asthma remedies he took they had no permanent effect. He had arranged to have ten treatments of Pleneurethic over a four-week period. Six months after the treatment terminated Frank said his asthma attacks had stopped except for one very mild and very short recurrence. Frank also said that the chronic heaviness in his forehead had also departed. He mentioned that his head seemed lighter and clearer. He also worked better at his job.

Frank received nothing from me other than the physical restructuring of the major spinal cord bioducts associated with the occipital foramen magnum and upper three cervical vertebrae. Ordinarily, more visits are scheduled for a case similar to his but we both wanted to see the effectiveness of a short series of corrections.

An interesting phenomenon which I call momentum was illustrated by Frank's case. Once the neural bioducts are properly treated and if the associated tissues are strong enough to hold, the brain and nerves will continue to regenerate long after the therapy procedures have terminated. Continued improvement following the discontinuance of treatment is called momentum. Momentum may be successfully established by a few visits in some cases. Other more difficult cases may require a year or more to bring them through the threshold into the free area of biological momentum which results from a substantial reversal of a bioductory malstructure.

It should be understood by now that chronically ill people uniformly have more than one problem which manifests itself in their chronic illness syndrome, and affects total health.

The following is a list of a number of salient features from individual cases:

A middle-aged man was complaining of progressive paralysis in his facial tissues. He was under care for extensive anatomical damage to his upper cervical bioducts. On one particular visit a treatment breakthrough occurred. Within seconds after the physical correction was made and the bioduct trauma was substantially removed from the nerve tracts of the central neural system transitting the duct, he felt a sharp pain proceed from the cervical nerve tissues and the bioductory area in question directly to his right ear.

The ear began to ache intensely and continued to ache on and off for several days. On his next visit the man commented that one of the earliest things he could recollect about his infancy was that he had a series of excruciating, nearly unbearable aches in his right ear. The man recognized his recent earaches as being a recurrence of the old ache he first noticed when he was a babe in swaddling clothes.

It is interesting to speculate about the origin of the bioduct injury in his upper cervical tissues. Could it have been the result of an early fall? Or was it perhaps due to a difficulty at birth which directed the heavy and presumptuous application of an obstetrician's steel clamps? Such clamps are sometimes used to almost maliciously jerk and twist a stubborn fetus from its position within an anesthetized and unconscious mother. In any case, early injury to the cervical neurological tissues caused the subsequent earaches and still later facial paralysis. Fortunately, although he was a definite candidate for crib death, it did not occur. As the earaches abated the facial paralysis commenced to disappear. All within a few days after the neural trauma had been reversed.

A woman of thirty had been experiencing the development of hideous splotches of red rash over various parts of her body. The rash would sometimes cover one side of her face. On other occasions it would appear on her neck and shoulder, and at other times it might cover large areas of her back and sides of her body. The rash would emerge, remain for a few days or weeks, and then dissipate only to reappear after a short interval.

The woman was accepted for treatment.

Nothing happened on the first few visits but on the fourth visit a heavy rash developed within seconds after she received therapy. The rash remained for several hours and then vanished. On her next visit the rash again appeared within seconds after correction of the neurological condition involved and vanished within a few hours. Her visits for the next month were characterized by the appearance followed by the disappearance of the rash within ever decreasingly short intervals of time. During the second month, the rash finally stopped appearing. To the date of writing, the woman has not suffered a reappearance of the rash. I might add that with the banishment of the rash the woman's anxiety and tension were also reduced. She became calm and obviously more enjoyable company for she married several months after the rash ceased to appear. Her whole person had improved.

She felt, however, that Pleneurethic had actually done nothing for her. She attributed her recovery to the man she had fallen in love with. She met him when on vacation about two months after she began to receive Pleneurethical treatment.

An extremely interesting incident occurred to the eyes of another middle-aged patient during the course of his Pleneurethical treatment. Since childhood he had been aware that the pupil of one eye was much larger than the pupil of the other eye. This person had a severe condition involving his upper cervical and upper thoracic bioducts. After several months of care, an exceptionally great step was made in bringing the affected bioducts into proper anatomical relationship and releasing pathological tension in the spinal cord and brain. Almost immediately afterward the pupils in both eyes assumed equal dimensions. This occurrence has a very logical explanation but it is excessively involved and beyond the scope of this work. Needless to say the person was receiving care for a condition far more serious than unmatched pupils. However, both conditions sprang from the same source and both were abolished when neurological integrity was restored.

The following case history was sent to me by a patient six months after I had treated her. When I first saw her I suggested she write down what she felt was wrong with her and the changes she noticed during the course of treatment and afterward. She is an American girl who was living in Thailand at the time of treatment.

February 21, 1968

As far back as five years ago I began to get a numb feeling on my left arm. I had a constant feeling of debility and was always feeling miserable. I seemed to be always depressed and often extremely so. I often flew into bad tempers. As well, I had a general feeling of being completely exhausted. I also felt insecure and was always scared about something.

I can only attribute these feelings to my being alone most of the time in a new and rather strange country and having only the children for company. I am trying to manage on my own and trying to learn the language. I also have to work full-time. To make it worse I have not made any friends here and my in-laws create problems.

Sometimes I have the compulsion to work nonstop until I am in a state of near collapse. After these periods I have terrible moods. It seems that the frustrations in my married life are accumulating. Coupled with very little rest and relaxation I am finding myself in an even more extreme state of nervousness. Three and a half years after having worked nonstop and having had a baby in between, I went on a three-week vacation, that was in mid-1966. I returned from that holiday feeling even more exhausted and in a worse nervous state than when I left.

For the first time in my life, during the latter part of that year I began to experience constant headaches. While I was away, I became very upset when I found that my lower gums had become so very swollen that I could hardly eat.

All of these things were followed by sleeplessness, which became worse over a five-week period. Everything was compounded by both domestic and other problems. From Christmas 1966 to the end of January 1967 I had hardly any sleep at all. I began to take sleeping pills, without prescription. In the beginning I took one pill a night but after about a month I increased the dose to four. But I still could not get any sleep. I would lie awake all night and be completely worn out by the morning. Even so, I kept going to work. I did everything practically automatically. By the time nightfall came I was wide awake again.

After approximately five to six weeks of going without sleep and trying to cope with a family and other problems, I became so tired with life in general that I tried to commit suicide. After this I went away for about five months to try to recuperate. I regained my appetite and after two months of rest I found that I was able to sleep properly again.

It was recommended that I should go to a psychiatrist and get my muddled mind straightened out but I never did. I felt I would only become more confused. Instead, I spent a few hours every week during those five months talking to Jesuit priests. I gained some valuable information from them. In July 1967 I returned home and rejoined my family. Shortly afterward I was again upset by domestic problems. Because of the physical conditions in the house where we lived I could not get enough sleep. The hot weather seemed to bother me and after a month I started to get headaches again. By September, I felt quite debilitated but I felt I could take the pressure. By December, I could hardly get any sleep. I had more headaches and I was very tense and I was given to crying fits.

Early in January 1968 I met a Pleneurethical person and was given an examination and a first treatment by him.

I did not see him for approximately two weeks after the first treatment. During those two weeks I was confined in hospital with what was diagnosed as German measles and a good case of "nerves." I was able to get some rest. The quiet in the hospital was very helpful and my fever disappeared. A week after I was discharged from the hospital I went for further Pleneurethical treatment.

Since that time he has given me six treatments, and I have experienced a number of improvements. I feel physically better in every way. I am more cheerful and contented with myself. I don't experience any attacks of the blues at all and I am not so easily upset. People say that I look much younger. I seem to be able to cope with the work in the office much better than I used to. I am also finding that I am not getting rattled when I have to work under pressure. I am in better command of myself and seem to be more self-confident. I think a lot faster and better. My thinking seems to be more lucid and I am not afraid any more. The constipation, which I suffered on and off for several years, is suddenly gone. My appetite is also much better.

The only problem I still have is sleeplessness. However, I must explain that I am living with my in-laws. The house is noisy. I now take about an hour to fall asleep and I wake up several times during the night. As a result I still feel tired in the morning.

Although it was explained to me that these are only temporary, I am experiencing pain in several spots on my back, below the base of my head, both sides, in the middle of my back, and below the waist. I also have shooting sensations on both sides of my head. Otherwise, I have never felt better, both physically and mentally, in the whole of my life.

February 24, 1968

In the last three days I have noticed further sensations and improvements. I am breathing easier, especially when I am lying down. Until very recently I never seemed to want to go to the Ladies' Room, for voiding purposes, like other women during the day. I now seem to be visiting it much more regularly and find myself going there about four or five times a day.

I used to suffer terrible nightmares and I am pleased to say that I have not been having any lately. All my dreams seem to be quite pleasant. I also seem to be sleeping better. In fact, I have slept well one out of the past three nights. Previously I used to go through a whole week without getting a good night's sleep.

It has also occurred to me that I did hurt my back a few years ago. Until now the incident had slipped my mind completely. I have been trying to recall when it was and how it happened but I cannot remember.

FEBRUARY 28, 1968

I was given another treatment on Monday, February 26. This time he seemed to have reached the bottom of my brains and touched the root of my troubles. As he reached what he called the suboccipital bioductory region, something big seemed to crack at the base of my head, on the left-hand side. Stinging sensations went from the base of my head in a diagonal direction down to the right-hand side of my back. I also felt shooting sensations going upward in all directions into my head. Then I felt something cool and a warm glow going all the way down to my feet. Suddenly the pain which was above the shoulders at the base of my head dissappeared.

For the first time in two years, after this experience I was able to sleep the moment I laid down. I had no dreams and woke up with a wonderful feeling of well-being. I slept well the next night which was rather unusual. Previously I slept well only for a night and very badly for the next three or four nights. When I did sleep I think it was only from complete exhaustion.

For the past few years I have also been waking up in the morning with swollen hands, but this seems to have stopped during the past two weeks.

In the approximately two months I was given treatment,

I have experienced a complete change of outlook and an overall improvement both mentally and physically.

The noise, people milling around, and the long hours in the office used to bother me to such an extent that I felt drained at the end of the day. I used to mope around all the time and be absorbed in self-pity with constant morbid thoughts. Now I can remain cheerful for days. Whereas I used to feel depressed for as long as a month, I now have only occasional slight attacks of the blues. I am able to throw these off in a very short time. I used to have a poor concentration. Now I am not so easily distracted. Since I have had treatment, the "butterflies" in my stomach have completely disappeared. I hardly seem to be afraid anymore. My outlook seems much more optimistic than in the past ten years or so.

* * *

The extent of Pleneurethical therapy is by no means limited to restructuring the bioductory system, although this chapter has focused exclusively upon this sector of Pleneurethical theory and practice. Restructuring the mentality can be equally significant in some cases. Mental restructuring will be dealt with in a subsequent volume. Pleneurethic employs its own unique technique in this interesting phase of the work. This work is devoted to healing the entire person.

9

THE "ETHIC"
IN PLENEURETHIC

PART 1

Pleneurethic, faithful to pure thought, endorses no religion, no special science, no politic. There are no priests in Pleneurethic, no sheep charged to follow its teachings on blind faith.

It does not menace government for control of the lives of people. It makes no alliance with officials of state. Pleneurethic's only alliance is individually with the persons constituting state. No one will be asked to contribute money for a temple building in the name of Pleneurethic. Each person builds his own, figuratively speaking, by enlightened thinking, good deeds, and considerate behavior without thought of reward.

Pleneurethic does not seek to preserve any civil establishment or social system. Nor does it seek to destroy.

Pleneurethic simply addresses itself to the task of bringing to the individual a personal sense of inner ethical well-being and comprehension of the rights of others. Once each person accepts responsibility for his own ethical upgrading, the quality of life generally will improve.

Pleneurethic bases morality on mind and the neural system.

That which is best for collective neural resources over the long term is good. That which unnecessarily harms the total neural establishment is bad.

The ethical outlook improves health potential because these cerebellar resources are constructively conserved. There is, therefore, a practical dividend to be derived from adoption of the ethical way.

Ethic is evaluated in terms of personal responsibility for constructive utilization of neural energy. The amount of such energy available to an individual is inelastic. It is nature's most precious resource.

Pleneurethic believes it is unethical to waste this resource or to conduct oneself in such manner as to cause waste of another's neural energy resources.

Brought to simplest terms, ethical behavior brings better economy of cerebellar energies than does unethical character. The ethical mind provokes less neurological turbulence than the unethical mind. It helps solve the inner energy crisis.

Thus, it is unethical to tangle deliberately the mental structure of another person with falsehood, depress it by demanding unnecessary occupation, destroy its symmetry and strength by damaging its organic abode, or obliterate it with a deadly device.

Yes, one of the most important aspects of Pleneurethic philosophy is individual acceptance of responsibility for ethical achievement. We are ethical not because some god commands it or because a churchman preaches it but because we ourselves, upon examining our own inner beings, want it and believe it necessary.

Thus, if we are unethical, it is because we have desired it so. We have hoodwinked or betrayed no one but ourselves.

If we place the ultimate authority for good conduct where it should be—on our own ethical shoulders—we immediately achieve a sobering insight into the realities of life on earth. We become more responsible citizens because we cannot shift the blame for our own failure to higher authority.

Life-styles that despoil life form, mislead mentality, and degrade the earth from which our material drape is drawn, are bad. They are unethical and antagonize the advance of civilization.

All life-styles are good that honor life forms, enlighten mentality, and revere its environment. Life-styles that constructively conserve vital capability and foster civilized well-being are good. They are Pleneurethical.

Ethic may be taught in the family, at school, in the civic auditorium, or army camp without mention of God, Buddha, Tao, or Mohammed. Pleneurethic provides a substantial foundation for instruction in ethic, based on personal integrity and devotion to high ethical principle. Supernatural figures accepted on faith need not be an ingredient of such teaching.

However, if any man needs a special God to believe in, for his own well-being, then by all means allow him to have his God. Attempts to deprive him of such belief conducive to his own comfort is improper.

By the same token, if there be a man who does not experience profit from belief in a special covenant with a gift-giving God, then it is wrong to inflict unusual burden upon him with a belief alien to his nature.

The Absolute, in the eyes of Pleneurethic, is believed to be immalleable to act or entreaty of man no matter how great man's worldly suffering. Man is a creature of the material world. He must look to things of this world and not the next for relief from worldly ills.

Pleneurethic believes that breach of universal law automatically results in illness or discomfort. Suffering is not the wrath of a jealous God but a predictable corollary of imprudent conduct with respect to the environment in which we must survive.

These consequences are impersonal and whatever discomfort we feel physically is not carried over into death. If there is a hell, it is here on earth and is with us constantly. It is not necessary to die to experience the forces of hell.

Hell is the result of being in disalignment with natural forces, and we begin to feel it the moment we deviate from consonance with physical and ethical law.

The concepts of heaven and hell are corollaries of a belief in a supernatural figure. Such concepts tend to destroy the assumption of personal responsibility for life. At the same time they serve to bulwark the indispensable posture of the clergy and perpetuate the costly church.

We are best advised to consider the future of civilization, rather than our own status in an obscure hereafter. Civilization is the highest achievement of humankind. As we ourselves aid this achievement so also are we blessed in equal portion.

Pleneurethic envisions civilization to be a living wheel of

majestic proportions rotating in evolution through space and time to its ultimate destiny.

And Pleneurethic finds it more relevant to put one's shoulder to the wheel and support its evolutionary advance than to pick up the cross to stamp out devils, burn witches, or draw and quarter infidels if they refuse conversion to the faith.

The wheel of civilization turns true on the structure of Pleneurethic as man considers what should be done rather than what could be done. The ethical distance between the possible and the desirable is vast indeed. Simply because something is feasible does not necessarily mean eternal good will result from that act.

A proper philosophy need not shift with changing culture. If a philosophy is correct, it remains as soundly applicable today as it did in the past and will continue so into the distant future.

Christian theology has indeed wavered over the years. Its opportunistic excesses are demonstrated when theologians shift their thinking on fundamental theology with the times.

Christian apologists now conjure a new God, a model for the 70s. The new Christian God, say these modernists, will not solve man's problems. He must solve them for himself!

Yes, theologians have definitely shifted their thinking. Now they endow their new God with characteristics markedly similar to Pleneurethic's Absolute.

Theologians are also on untenable ground when they speak of spiritual cure of chronic physical illness.

Pleneurethic grants them freedom to advocate spiritual cure of spiritual sickness, but when they step over into the temporal world and imply that spiritual sickness causes chronic physical and mental illnesses, they draw argument.

Pleneurethic professes no quarrel with religion in the sense that it provides a basis for ethical behavior. It does, however, question the assumption that only through organized church religion can a sense of morality be developed in the individual.

Conversion to and embracement of ethic, Pleneurethic sees hopefully as a process occurring within the individual—not through imposition of an external code prescribed by churchmen upon the individual.

Pleneurethic believes that the law of the universe is not depraved and since man has emerged from the fabric of that law, man likewise is not depraved.

In the Pleneurethical universe all that is good is of our making and all that is evil is also created by us. This universe contains neither good nor evil but a system of forces that furnishes the constituents for our earthly bodies and within which we as individuals must exist.

Our potential for exercise of free will provides us with option for choice depending on our experience, our degree of ignorance or illumination, and our goal. With free will comes opportunity to interpret events as good or evil according to the structure of our mentality.

Good is synonymous with life in complete accordance with universal forces. Evil is synonymous with the misery and calamity that accompanies conduct transgressing universal forces.

Evil comes from activity of man. It does not spring from the presence of universal forces. Moreover, evil is an abstraction and an invention of man, not of the universe. Man's evil is neither good nor bad in the eye of universal forces. So-called evil simply is manifestation of the result of man's infringement of that force. Evil is bad in the eyes of man because it is a painful reminder of man's inharmonious collision with forces of the universe.

Deep, pure, and genuine interest in the welfare of all life about us is the basis for Pleneurethical conduct.

The true guide to proper social actions cannot be found through intellectual observance of theistic commandments or religious canon. It can be found only through vigilant inspection and cultivation of one's own ultrallect and a firm desire to live harmoniously with life about us.

Each individual is a living result of the forces at play in our universe. As such, each individual has the seeds of grace and divinity within himself. His chief task, then, is to identify the seeds and cultivate them.

Each must look within himself for the spark of ethical greatness. Each is responsible to himself for his own actions. Whatever suffering he experiences is a direct result of abandonment, in one way or another, of this basic responsibility. No other individual— priest, analyst, counselor, father, mother, brother, sister, or judge —can set aside or usurp this responsibility.

Pleneurethic promises no cozy abode in the spiritual hereafter, nor threatens a home in hell for failure to abide by certain dictates.

Rather an individual's thoughts and deeds are tallied immediately within himself. Consequences are summarily rendered and immediately faced by him.

Pleneurethic is philosophy for rational man, for reasonable man. It seeks to foster and perpetuate in each individual an unquenchable desire to lead the ethical life on earth.

There is, also, a purely practical dividend to be derived from adherence to the ethical way. The ethical outlook improves health potential. Why? Because neural resources are constructively conserved.

Ethic, then, is the final goal of Pleneurethic—ethic of spontaneous buoyant nature arising from deep inner ethical resolve.

PART 2

The intelligent man does not misuse his own cerebellar resources and the ethical man does not abuse those of others. The wise man, through his understanding, is both intelligent and ethical. He knows the futility of endeavoring to break the law of the Absolute. The only thing broken in the process is the man who essays it, or those permissive persons who encourage it through inaction.

The rule of ethic is Pleneurethic's most cherished shibboleth.

In Pleneurethic, ethic is not limited to being provincially based on a regionally recognized deity. Rather, it is based on a more universal and perpetual principle. That is, the conservative and constructive use of civilization's neural energy resources.

Pleneurethic's concept of brain capability translates into all the affairs of man. It even provides an eternally irrefrangible basis for ethical life. This base is firm and measurable—something that such concepts as love or divine spirits or holy ghosts are not.

The rule of ethic yields a comprehensible standard which cannot be legitimately brushed aside by willful persons seeking their own selfish ends. When these ends are wrapped up in achieving competency and skill to selfishly manipulate other people to their detriment, the rule of ethic is disserved.

Pleneurethic is the strictest of all philosophies and religions. It puts each person on his own responsibility for the successful completion of his ultimate destiny. He alone is responsible for locating and discovering, developing and manifesting his own ethical wisdom.

The penalties in Pleneurethic are great. So are the rewards. Conversely, when ethical maturity is achieved there are neither penalties nor rewards.

Pleneurethicists shoulder the full responsibility for their thought and behavior. They do not allow themselves the luxury of excusing their ethical lapses by transferring the responsibility for their errant conduct to any other person. Pleneurethicists are not saved by a god or excused by priests. Neither are they offered any pink and frilly refuge because they were allegedly discriminated against in youth by some vague caprice of society. They cannot plead extenuating circumstances if they commit felonious acts while they are ill or intoxicated. Illness does not permit any person to act either outrageously or unethically. If a person is truly ethical he will be so regardless of whether he is sick or well. Abuse by others does not grant a person the license to be ruthless and unethical. Each man must make his own way, abiding by all ethical rules and intentionally molesting no one. If a person cannot reach the goal he wants to achieve, then, rather than become despondent, he must either revise it or else discipline himself to the point where he can achieve it.

The greatest wisdom lies in the decision to live by truth as it is found in eternal ethic. Ethical truth shields and protects, and so does acting in a spirit of goodwill which allows a person to give more than he takes. At the same time it lets him act as he believes. Too often today covert belief and overt talk and behavior are dissimilar. This leads to a stifling of true communication between people and inspires hateful distrust and promotes fearful concern.

Such dissimilarity also frustrates civilization when certain persons give lip service to law, but live capriciously outside its edicts—so they can better capitalize on predictable and orderly citizenry.

Pleneurethic provides a balancing pivot of ethic around which law and justice may ultimately merge. Rule of ethic in fact transcends the rule of law and the imposition of justice, yet embraces them both. Rule of justice versus the rule of law has been the basis of schism in civilization since men grouped themselves in societies, governed by a rule of law.

If the law is properly formed and correctly applied, justice for all will prevail. But if law is improper because it is archaic, or unreasonably favors some special interest group, there can be no justice. Even if law is proper, but is incorrectly applied by unethical men, there will again be a breach of justice.

Law then, through its application, may conflict with justice because law tends to become rigid, barren, and remote from the realities of life. It becomes, alternately, excessively strict or uselessly permissive. Justice, on the other hand, tends to become a flighty thing, blown on the winds of individual interpretation. Even the courts may violate justice for the body politic, while they foster increasing irresponsibility for minor wrongdoers by issuing only token sentences.

There should be a common ground where law and justice meet. There should be a central standard which law and justice can jointly embrace. Throughout history there have been many efforts to achieve such a balance. Christianity, for example, has for the last 2,000 years claimed to provide both a basis for law and a refuge for those seeking justice. This basis is provided by Christianity's religious canon: faith in God and obedience of His commandments as interpreted by theologians, ministers of the Gospel, and all others wishing to quote their favorite biblical text plucked from a host of sections which tend to contradict one another.

Pleneurethic forms a stable base, of universal application, to all people throughout the world who seek justice. Through Pleneurethic, the world can achieve a new level of civilization. Application of its principles will release a potential for creativity never before enjoyed by the world. A resurgence of eternal ethic powered by increased mental competency will surely uplift civilization.

Pleneurethic includes both a thrust for quality of life through its advocacy of ethic, and a bulwark for quantity of life by virtue of its method of restoring total brain capability.

Its application can bring a reign of reason to a troubled, confused, struggling world. A world whose civilization is splintered along religious lines, fractured by nationalism and consumed by disintegration of thought when it should be united on basic issues and problems.

Reconstruction of world civilization in a manner more in harmony with the reality of life is the aim of Pleneurethic. This is possible because there does exist a universal factor in life, which, when applied to a restructuring of world civilization, can improve it.

Pleneurethic recognizes this universal factor in life. It integrates thought. It believes in eternal ethic as opposed to the ethic of expediency and exposes itself in selfless high idealism.

The ethic of Pleneurethic is related to the structure of the mentality and to brain competence. An evil and sinful mentality imposes a heavy brain burden both on others and the person possessing it. An ethical mentality, on the other hand, uplifts the level of brain competence and elevates its energetic buoyancy.

Since Pleneurethic postulates health is derived from overall neurological competence, it follows that the ethical mentality improves chances for health and success in life. Evildoing inflicts people with weighty neurological encumbrances, decreasing their chances for health and creative productivity.

This is the basis for the Pleneurethical postulate that ethic and morality influence the levels of health an individual or civilization enjoys.

The structure of the mentality mobilizes the forces of a

vibrant brain and funnels it into a pattern of personal behavior and predisposes the possessor to a life ranging from hostility and bitter recrimination and assassination to sympathetic understanding and helpfulness and ethical character.

Malstructures of the mentality can be shifted, reinforced, or removed by manipulation of the mental structure. The structure of mentality is impregnable to alteration on some occasions and in other circumstances it is flexible without limitations.

Those responsible for the development of a child should help it from the very beginning to develop an ethically structured mentality from the Pleneurethical viewpoint.

Ethic is concerned with those basic beliefs which constitute the hard-core mental structures of character and make up the basis for an individual's habitual conduct. It is also concerned with those superficial beliefs that let the individual change his overt conduct but not his habitual thinking and real inner character. Beliefs which are considered ethical are either felt to be good in themselves or because they constitute the means to a proper end. Conduct which is unethical is either not good in itself or leads to a bad end. The consequences of beliefs or acts must be considered if they are to be labeled good or bad.

Ethic is the finest achievement of mentality and provides the basis for social law and order. Ethic would seem to include more than intelligence. It seems to indicate a high quality of mentation concerning the good of society; whereas intelligence alone, no matter how quantitatively brilliant, is apt to be self-seeking, egocentric, and even perhaps antisocial. Intelligence is more a quantity, and ethic more a quality, of thought, at least from the vantage of society as a whole in its need for law and order.

Ideal character cannot be developed by memorizing moral codes, but people with ideal characters have developed the ethical insight which allows them to construct moral codes at will to fit every occasion. They possess empathy for ethic.

The source of ethic is the desire to survive, and to aid the survival of the species. It springs from a heartfelt wish to live amongst people, helping them and understanding their needs and aiding their survival. Even though the society in which we live is competitive there are ethical guidelines which establish limits of force or device to be sanctioned in ethical competitive endeavor. Therefore, we do not kick people when they are down, nor do we endeavor to outsmart the blind, the moronic, the totally defeated, or those who are not as gifted as ourselves. We sincerely strive to be intellectually honest.

Absolute ethic, a phrase coined by Pleneurethic, means an ethic based on eternal values and on belief and conduct which enhances the preservation and proper evolution of our species as well as the proper cultivation of the entire living community. It is not the ethic of expediency. Absolute ethic is as intricate as absolute law and can never be laid out in a fully complete and polished written code. The final authority for moral obligation springs from a person's own ethical consciousness. Pure ethic is an ideal, never achieved by anyone. Yet a sense of eternal ethic exists in everyone, even if it is imperfectly manifested in behavior. Pleneurethists believe there is an absolute ethic which provides an absolute rule for good conduct. If it is drawn on, it can result in optimum cerebellar competency both for the individual and for our species en masse.

Two of Pleneurethic's few slogans are:

Give your life to your better self. Consult your better self for the answers to life's problems and strive earnestly throughout the succeeding days to achieve it.

10

PLENEURETHIC

PART 1

Pleneurethic is based on pure structural science rather than mystery or metaphysics or how well a remedy lends itself to commercialization. It is the newest of the various life philosophies. I conceived it in August 1963 after a lengthy and arduous period of research.

Among other things it was the first school to discriminate clearly between acute and chronic illness based upon the symmetry of the brain and related structures.

One of the most significant achievements of Pleneurethic was that it allowed potentially chronic brain damage to be accurately diagnosed and distal causes corrected, thus forestalling the structural deterioration of central neurological tissues which result in serious mental and physical breakdowns.

By putting brain requirements at the axis of its philosophy I integrated the art of healing and the science of healing, and provided a rational basis for a better philosophy of life. I therefore organized a proper healing philosophy and established a practical school of diagnosis and therapy grounded in pure structural science.

I created Pleneurethic because I felt there was a need for more truth in the world and less chicanery. I felt that the major mental and physical problems of the chronically sick were not due to a pinched nerve in a lateral spinal foramen, nor a sinful wish, nor even a germ or a repressed hatred, although charlatans were growing rich making people think they were.

The most important incidents in the development of Pleneurethic were discovering other theories and practices which did not work as they were claimed to work particularly in the treatment of

207

chronic illness. This was especially true of the religious, holy, or evil spirit approach. Repressed psychological conflict in the alleged unconscious mind from childhood due to nebulous events, or spirit hostility just do not cause chronic illness. A repressed psychological hatred deep in the conscious mind may cause an acute tightness in the stomach when the hatred surfaces, but it does not have the power to cause chronic organic pathology or chronic mental illness.

The various psychotherapeutic schools also seemed inadequate when they declared that the cause of chronic depression or hyper-irritability was due to either grief or repressed anger at someone near and dear. The theory does not hold up in the face of the facts. These are that the loss of loved ones or repressed anger and guilt thoroughly depress some persons and fail to affect others very much at all. Thus, these psychotherapeutic schools, in my mind, fall into the same category as the germ proponents. Not every person catches a cold when near a person with a cold. Only those susceptible catch colds and susceptibility is a product of brain problems.

Neither do all persons suffer mental torment if they flout moral strictures. Hellfire religion appears notoriously deficient in explaining a good many things which must be rationally explained if a philosophy is to be universally accepted.

Pleneurethic finally emerged when I realized after a lifetime of searching and testing, that brain was the prime and axial structure for realistically interrelating the various aspects of the total human being. No one before Pleneurethic had satisfactorily accounted for the multitude of seemingly paradoxical or unexplainable occurrences in the human being. However, many events in the body and mind can now be easily explained by Pleneurethic principles and extensive projections from its basic presumptions.

Once I achieved that primary breakthrough in my thinking, after decades of intense investigation, other breakthroughs followed. I then proceeded to expound my views, vigorously and fearlessly, as follows:

* Restate anatomy and physiology, pathology and psychology, from the standpoint of brain structure and symmetry.

* Postulate that chronic disease can be caused by accumulations of structural distortion manifesting mental and physical symptoms concurrently.

* Discriminate between acute and chronic illness both mental and physical on the basis of brain involvement.

* Identify a new system of the human body, namely the bioductory system.

* Explain the idea that chronic distortions to the bioductory system structure install chronic disturbance to brain structure and alter the range of its biological function, affect bodily content, and cause chronic diseases of infinite variety.

* Describe the anatomy of the psyche, and forecast that mental perceptions of reality or truth are influenced by changes in brain structure both micro and macro.

* Erect the concept of the chronic anxiety syndrome, showing its relationship to brain distortion.

* Advocate that brain and mind are separate although closely interrelated tissues, and destroy the Freudian concept that chronically abnormal behavior stems from psychological conflict repressed into the unconscious mind by frustrations in childhood.

* Note the correlation between chronic inability to relax because of chronic brain tension and the incidence of degenerative and other chronic diseases.

* Correlate chronic brain illness with criminality, atypical behavior, unemployability, and frayed nerves that require relief through alcohol and drugs.

* Show daydreams and night dreams as a device to reduce brain tension due to events of the days before. Reveal relationships between nightmares and atypical behavior during chronic illness caused by chronic brain problems.

* Override the idea that a pinched spinal nerve in the lateral

foramen causes chronic illness, and overcome the food fad
approach to chronic illness.

* Expound an absolute source of all force as opposed to
irrational deities supposed to be capable of inflicting illness
as vengeance for real or imagined sin.

* Show that sin is not a cause of chronic illness but that
chronic illness can cause a vague but nevertheless very
intense feeling of guilt.

* Develop a theory of ethic and truth based on economy of
neural energy, and on the structure of the brain.

* Show that malstructures of mentality, from intellectual
conflict and unresolved problems in the conscious mind,
depress brain capability perceptibly and acutely.

* Profess health to be a product of brain vigor and stability.

The axial notion of Pleneurethic is the belief that total
brain capability establishes parameters of reality for the individual,
and is a legitimate standard of evaluation long overlooked by
philosophers and researchers. We are not made chronically sick
by germs, pinched peripheral nerves, repressed wishes or a ma-
levolent godly spirit. Rather, we are made chronically ill by
processes which chronically reduce, distort, or destroy brain
capability, brain fidelity, and brain structure.

Some rudiments of Pleneurethic were already in existence
before I began to develop my theory. I learned much from
studying the basic works on anatomy, physiology, psychology,
and religion. But, after the best part of a lifetime spent in searching
for answers, I was disappointed with what I found already in print.
Moreover, much of what I read was in error.

PART 2

Through intensive study and inquiry into the various healing
methods it became obvious that the least understood forms of
illness throughout the ages have been those of the chronic variety.

Mature people know what causes most complaints. They
always have. But the cause of long-standing chronic conditions

that grow worse with time, eventually incapacitating and then totally destroying their victims, has remained a mystery. The course of the disease is seldom the same in a variety of cases. It is sometimes rapid and sometimes unmercifully slow and seems to tantalize or punish the afflicted. An expert in torture could hardly impose more agony than some forms of chronic illness which can snuff out the life of a child at the age of seven or allow it to struggle through a lifetime of pathology to die in its fifties, sixties, or seventies.

The effects of the disease on the personality can be so horrendous that victims in the long past have submitted to trephining operations carried out on the head with a wooden hammer and stone chisel to gain relief. In other places they have allowed themselves to be hung over open fires and willingly submitted to terrifying encounters with medicine men whose tools of the trade are evil-colored smoke, vile-tasting fluid, and incantations. And in our own society victims are only too willing to try anything that might bring them physical or mental relief. Thus, they are, and always have been, easy prey for any charlatan. And there are as many charlatans in our modern hospital as most any place else. Vicious use of X rays and many damaging chemicals are cases in point.

One of the more prominent concepts of the cause of chronic disease, prevalent throughout healing history, has been that of spirits. Mankind has, since its primitive beginnings, been obsessed with various forms of hostile spirits as a cause of misery and chronic suffering and the use of good spirits to combat evil spirits.

Thus, he has used witch doctors, sorcerers, priests, and holy men in an attempt to evict evil from afflicted bodies.

The notion that bacteria (a microscopic plant) caused chronic disease was a solid step away from the earlier idea that a mysterious force of supernatural origin was to blame. Moreover, because bacteria is physical, it was alleged that it was best combated with a material agency. This agency, a chemical, manufactured in the innermost recesses of the chemist's alcove, would clean the ailing body of its awesome invader—the bacteria.

But when the bacteria refused to be cleansed away by corrosive drugs and the patient remained disgustingly and chronically sick, the bacteria was awarded the property of being able to miraculously change its characteristics to thwart drugs touted as invincible. When the body still ailed of some unknown thing and unfortunately died of it after all of the bacteria in it had been killed the blame was flung onto viruses.

Therapy aimed at the mind is said to be able to cure degenerative physical illness which occurs where no microorganism can be found. However, the effectiveness of psychiatry in curing degenerative mental and physical illness has been patently and pathetically inadequate. Despite the resources plowed into it in the form of highly trained men, the principle upon which psychiatry is founded is faulty as far as the treatment of chronic disease is concerned.

This is mainly because psychiatry is based on the philosophical postulate that a disease which cannot be cured by drugs comes from the mind. Too often when chronic illness sufferers fail to respond to psychiatric treatment, the cause of their suffering is labeled as psychosomatic and secreted away in a fairyland called the unconscious mind.

Pleneurethic claims that psychiatry is confused and guessing at the facts when it postulates and discusses the unconscious mind.

The main confusion lies in the erroneous idea that memories, which at one time were on the surface of the conscious mind and later penetrated deeper into it from years of misuse and repression, can harm the brain enough to be the principal cause of chronic mental and physical illness.

Psychiatry is not alone in its failure to come to grips with the cause of chronic illness. Every form of healing appears to skirt around the problem and attempts to relate its cause to factors relating to acute illness rather than attempting to classify chronic illness into a class of its own. This is the main reason, I believe, why the cause of incurable degenerative physical and mental illness remained a mystery and resulted in so much confusion and heartbreak.

Healers were almost right when they dismissed many of the symptoms of chronic illness as being "all in the mind."

I contend that the cause of chronic degenerative mental and physical illness comes not from the mind but instead from actual brain trauma resulting from bioductory system distortions in the regions close to the head, neck, and shoulders.

These distortions are caused by a particular type of accident, which could have resulted in death from brain injuries if the brain had not been protected by the bioductory system. This system can be extensively damaged and, when the damage is severe, distortions to its anatomical structure occur.

The bioductory system is the system of ducts that are supposed to protect the brain and its spinal extension from physical injury.

It surrounds the nerves in the spine and forms both osseous and soft tissue ducts through which the nerve tracts pass. It directly supports, shields, and aids the neural system. Therefore, it is one of the most important anatomical structures in the body. Before Pleneurethic it was one of the least understood. In fact, its existence as a system was not even recognized. It is so important to life that I called it the bioductory system.

Moderate or light physical trauma to the body does not harm much of anything at all. But heavy physical trauma such as an injury at birth, a severe automobile whiplash, athletic field injury, a fall on the head and neck from a tree or horseback may cause the part of the bioductory system just under the head, in the neck, or across the shoulders to be so extensively traumatized that it cannot return to normal.

The fact that it is extensively injured is often slowly reflected back into the central neural system on which it imposes a direct mechanical strain. This chronic stress, added to other tensions of everyday life, reflects into the mind and repercusses into the body to create havoc. This havoc is compounded because the brain is unable to pinpoint the source of the damage.

The bioductory system is susceptible to an infinite variety of traumatization patterns. The resulting pattern of damage to the brain is determined by the specific structural mechanics of bioductory derangement. It is, therefore, difficult to list all of the points upon which bioductory diagnosis hinges simply.

But basically almost any chronic stiffness along the back, neck, head, or hips denotes damage to some sector of the bioductory system. Sometimes the sufferer notices only a headache, a painful jaw that locks on occasion, pressure at the base of the head, yellowish or bloodshot eyes, or perhaps bursitis with subsequent arthritis in the fingers.

Some nightmares, sleeplessness, fitful sleep schedules, or mental instabilities are indicative of chronic brain damage from bioductory system problems. Chronic anger is also a symptom which may indicate bioductory system damage.

Since chronic bioductory system trauma, especially in the head, neck, and shoulder areas, causes varying degrees of chronic brain damage, there will be chronic symptoms occurring concurrently both in the mind as mental illness and in the body as organic disorder. This explains such mysterious conditions as hysteria and psychosomatic illnesses where both mental and physical illness go hand in hand.

Many chronic illness sufferers are unable to be definite about their complaints. They will be vague and prone to change their story about their illness from day to day and year to year. If the sufferer had only an acute complaint stemming from a broken arm, a bruised muscle, or a broken and aching tooth he would be very specific about its presence and location. But a patient suffering from a bioductory system disorder will complain of an unending variety of symptoms. The physician is hard pressed to gather the symptoms together coherently enough to label them with a specific disease name.

To make matters worse there is no observable reason for the person to be ill, nor is there anything patently evident for family or friends to recognize as a valid cause for illness. Thus, people tend to lose their patience with a person who is chronically ill, especially when the illness drags on for years with characteristic periods of exacerbations and remissions. Unable to convince anyone that he is really ill, the victim feels rejected, misunderstood, unneeded, unwanted, and resentful. He will often consider suicide or demand needless exploratory surgery in a fruitless effort to convince others that he is really ill.

Actually, his condition is so serious that if it is not corrected it will kill him. As the condition worsens bacteria of various types, depending on the location and nature of the tissue breakdown which invariably follows bioductory damage, begin to appear.

One of the main reasons why the cause and treatment of chronic illness has remained a mystery over the centuries is because scholars and philosophers failed to take a structural approach to it. The truth of the matter, therefore, eluded them. They also failed to gather isolated symptoms into a logical pattern, and then find the central cause of the pattern which could be treated.

The Pleneurethical approach toward the healing of chronic illness and restoring cerebellar sufficiency is fundamentally a structural approach. It is applied on the intellectual and ethical levels as well as on the physical level. The concept of structure is not mutually exclusive to Pleneurethic. In order to comprehend the idea of structure it should be associated with function and content.

The idea of content and its interrelationship with structure and function was instrumental in inspiring such healing approaches as medicine and surgery. Thus, in medicine some ingredients are added to the body in a bid to improve its content, thereby beneficially modifying the body's function and microstructure. Surgery, on the other hand, removes content from the body which has hopelessly deteriorated into fulminating inflammation, purulence, and ulcers. The nutritional approach to healing is also based on the concept of content. It attempts to modify the body's structure and function by shifting the nutritional content.

The basic idea of content and its ability to change structure and function is very simple. Yet there are definite limits to which content modification will be able to shift the body's structure and function relationships. These limits are severely attenuated in one direction and not the other. Thus, if we totally restrict nutritional intake ino a healthy body, structure and function will be completely repealed by a process called death within a period of time. However, revision of content intake through dietary improvement will definitely not create health in those chronic cases where sickness is due to basic gross or macrostructural problems. That which is true of limitations on healing with the nutritional approach is likewise true with medicine and surgery.

Content availability controls the structural design and if the content of the structure is improper the structure will be degeneratively influenced and its function negatively affected.

Several current healing disciplines and philosophies believe content to be the only approach to healing. They are wrong in this philosophical assumption and that is why they have not found a true cure for chronic illness.

Let us review an example which shows how improper structure or structural abnormalities can prevent function and unbalance content.

Suppose we have a stream which moves fast and true through a well-structured stream bed. Its watery content is clear and its function of draining the land is unimpeded. Now suppose a landslide changes the structure of the stream bed. The water no longer flows properly. The flow is sluggish and the content of the stream is filled with sludge and debris. Sediment is deposited and dark treacherous marshy areas develop which are filled with bacteria, insects, slime, and other low forms of life. The function of the stream to drain the land is destroyed. The soil sickens and only coarse forms of vegetation prevail through the readaptation of life to the new unclean environment. Slime forms and grows out of control.

And so it is with the human body when the basic bioductory structure is seriously disarranged. The content is degraded and the body functions are revised negatively.

As the body's function and content are revised because of the deteriorating structure, many things occur. Flesh, once vigorous and responsive, becomes turgid and of low quality. Areas of extreme tissue deterioration are walled off in saclike pouches. The low-grade areas occasionally break down into occasional sores, especially if they are involuntarily pressed to accomplish work. Cells grow out of control in certain areas because neurological communication has been lost.

In order to meet the changing chemical content of our body due to structural modification, the tissue cells revise their shape. The properties of the cells change, because their content has shifted due to unbalanced chemical content environment. In the final years or months of life, peculiarly shaped cells that may appear as foreign invaders are given such names as cancer. Such cells are not foreign but merely a living readaptation of normal cells as a result of the deteriorating chemical content of the body caused initially by structural abuse to the bioductory system and to the brain.

This chronic disease process can be arrested and reversed by Pleneurethical therapy. All traces of cancerous symptoms can be removed if corrective therapy is begun before irreversible brain changes set in.

Structure is the category which dictates content requirement and functional capability. If structure fails, both content and function will be jeopardized in an infinite variety of inimical ways.

Efforts to save the structure, which has been disorganized through traumatic force, will fail if the only avenues of therapy are by way of content replenishment and functional stimulation. Unless the basic structural disorder which began the degenerative trend is corrected no cure can be achieved on a permanent basis.

Pleneurethic is a structural approach oriented toward the basic structures of our bodies on several levels. It contends that chronic physical structural disorders respond only to cures of a physical nature. Acute intellectual structural disorders can only be corrected by intellectual methods. Ethical malstructures are best corrected through a meditative approach. Such is the essence of Pleneurethic.

PART 3

In advancing the rationale of Pleneurethic, the author realizes he opposes many existing philosophies of life and healing. Therefore, he is obligated not only to present his own theories but to indicate why he disagrees with the philosophy of others. These expressions of disagreement are not directed against any individual but solely against the philosophy represented by opposing schools.

Pleneurethic is irrevocably dedicated to the idea that the only effective method of treating the whole person and of controlling chronic illness is reliance on the restoration of the structure and function of brain.

This is predicated on the conviction that the cause of chronic physical and mental illness lies in the physics of anatomical structure precipitating chronic brain disturbance reinforced acutely by stresses generated by mental malstructures and toxic pollutants entering the bloodstream.

One of the earliest concepts of the cause of chronic illness in healing history was that of evil spirits. Mankind, since primitive times, has been obsessed with the idea of hostile spirits as a cause of misery and chronic suffering.

Early man had his witch doctors and sorcerers to frighten away evil spirits. In the Middle Ages, man resorted to intervention by priests to alter the impact of revengeful spiritual forces thought to cause chronic illness. Prayer and laying on of hands were among the remedies advanced to seek redress. Modern man still has his priest who is believed to be an effective medium for dispelling discomfort and curing illnesses such as cancer.

The idea that bacteria (a microscopic plant) caused chronic illness was a solid step away from the Middle Ages and its concept of supernaturalism. Bacteria, having physical properties, were thought to be best combated by a material agency—hence, the development of chemicals manufactured in the chemist's alcove.

When bacteria failed to be dispersed with use of corrosive drugs, medical science pointed to the virus, so small it cannot be seen with the average microscope, and, since it is not really alive, it cannot be killed! Thus was it possible to explain the enigma of a body in which all bacteria were seemingly destroyed by chemicals or drugs yet in which chronic illness persisted.

Pleneurethic asserts modern medicine to be academically provincial when, after claiming total therapeutic competence, it narrows its view to chemistry. The medical world is grossly unscientific when it insists on constricting the scope of its search to correlating symptoms of chronic illness with the presence of virus and bacteria. Myopic preoccupation with the tools of trade—the microscope and the test tube—has led medical academicians down a false trail.

Pathological levels of bacteria or viruses connected with chronic illness and disease do not flourish in the healthy body. The number of bacteria present in any given tissue multiplies to become chronically and pathologically evident only when the body has lost its ability to resist or to repair itself; in short, when there is pathological deficiency of neurological stimulation from depleneurization of brain tissue.

The crime of modern medicine is not so much its exclusive preoccupation with bugs and chemicals as it is in the specious claims of offering a complete health service, in the use of the public communications media to foster an untrue image, in failure to explore legitimate avenues leading to the cure of chronic illness, in prevention of congenital disorders in progeny born to parents with certain forms of chronic disease, and in the careless use of chemical and radiation techniques which ultimately prove to be worse than the original affliction.

Medicine's endeavor to discover the source of chronic disease, by restricting its search to correlating isolated chronic illness symptoms with the presence of foreign microscopic invaders, is on the same level of short-sightedness as studying the movement of wind with reference to a single mountain and neglecting the overall relationship of total air movement systems on the surface of the earth.

In Pleneurethic, the chronically ill person promises to become as much a study in physical and electronic stress as in chemical imbalance.

Healing is partially lifted from the College of Chemistry to the College of Physics. In fact, the College of Physics has no vested interest or philosophical hang-up on chemical dosage as a cure for chronic illness. Rather, physics understands structure and stress, ducts and distortion, and patterns of functional collapse correlated with patterns of structural disruption.

Pleneurethic does not deny the existence of toxic chemical pressures on the neural system in chronic cases but these chemical pressures, Pleneurethic contends, are secondard and simply augment the primary cause. Hence, drug therapies addressed to overcoming these secondary pressures are ineffective. They do not cure chronic illness. They simply palliate some symptoms.

Biochemistry at this twentieth-century juncture has one giant defect. It cannot point to the first cause of biochemical imbalance in the chronically ill body. It can, for instance, determine an insufficiency of insulin, but biochemical testing by itself cannot indicate the prime cause of that insufficiency. Therefore, prescription of insulin is not curative but constitutes a temporary expedient at best.

Philosophers of healing are faced with a basic problem: does alteration of biochemistry constitute the cause of illness or is an altered biochemistry the result of a more basic cause?

If we conclude that fortuitous alterations of biochemical content are the prime source of disease, then the proper remedy is correction of the disorganized biochemistry by adding necessary biochemicals in proper amount. This is the line of action now pursued by modern drug doctors.

Others, embracing another philosophy, believe that biochemical upset in the body is caused by germs. The cure in either case is thought to be a drug that will either kill the invading germs without killing surrounding body cells or neutralize the germ products that allegedly upset proper biochemical balance.

Pleneurethical philosophy advocates the cause of chronic chemical imbalance associated with chronic disease to be caused by brain problems. Hence, remedy is to be addressed to that axial region.

The present era of commercial drug medicine began in the nineteenth century. Medicine is now largely under control of the gigantic pharmaceutical industry.

The profit in drugs is fantastic. They are easily and rapidly dispensed, and a new drug can be put on the market complete with total advertising build-up in a matter of weeks.

The best that medicine can do for many chronic degenerative ailments is to reduce the severity of symptoms. At the same time, the main course of the basic chronic affliction continues to degenerate, unchanged by pharmacy.

Pharmacists have discovered and produced lotions, salves, and antiseptics that hasten the healing of acute wounds. Their stimulants have saved lives threatened by severe, acute trauma. Heart stimulants, vasoconstrictors, and various other drugs are splendid additions to the storehouse of knowledge possessed by modern-day medicine. Pharmacy does reduce somatic pain, temporarily relieve mental stress, and restore tranquility for a time. But, Pleneurethic contends, none of these drugs will reverse the course of the chronic disease process by correcting its cause.

Many concepts of healing are based on mechanical operations. Surgery is a mechanical procedure. Massage, whirlpool baths, vibratory tables—all devices are within this range.

Acupuncture is a surgical form of nerve goading. Highly irritative and stimulative, even to the point of insensitivity, it requires a fine knowledge of neural anatomy.

Persons practicing acupuncture are to be applauded for their logic in associating a chronically sick organ with its faulty innervating nerve tract.

However, their therapy is not of a basic nature, Pleneurethic believes, because it does not correct the cause of the chronic nerve problem. By goading the nerve they admittedly stimulate it to renewed vigor, but such stimulation is of an impermanent nature. It soon reverts to its former condition of apathy.

Yes, nerve goading by acupuncture practitioners and improper joint manipulation by random method may temporarily excite nerves. But this brief period of well-being is likely to be followed by an accelerated neural deterioration.

Psychiatry, a major subschool of medicine, frequently explains degenerative mental or physical illness as a product of psychological conflict in the unconscious mind. The treatment, therefore, should be mental—not chemical.

There is serious confrontation between the claims of psychiatry and the claims of Pleneurethic about the cause and cure of chronic illness. Many psychiatrists, medical doctors, and religionists have insisted on a mental cure for chronic mental illness. Pleneurethic believes chronic mental illness to be a brain problem due primarily to a physical cause—not an unconscious repression, chemical, or spiritual cause, although toxic pollutants or psychological stresses may intensify the chronic mental condition.

Pleneurethic claims psychiatry is confused when it postulates and discusses the unconscious mind. Memories that at one time were on the surface of the conscious mind and later penetrated deeper because of years of disuse and repression do not harm the brain sufficiently to be principal causes of chronic mental and physical illness. These memories, Pleneurethic contends, are not and never were in an unconscious area of the mind!

Thus, psychiatry's theory that chronic degenerative illness comes from the so-called unconscious mind is untenable. Instead, Pleneurethic sees it as the result of actual brain trauma due to bioductory distortions, especially those more cephalward.

In certain types of insanity science has found a malbiochemistry in the brain. This malbiochemistry, Pleneurethic believes, is not the first cause of the insanity, nor are the germs or viruses that may or may not be present. If we treat either or both medically, we will relieve symptoms only. The prime cause of the brain's deterioration—depleneurization—will remain unchecked.

Pleneurethic carries no brief against psychology or psychotherapy in general. Both of these fields have made contributions to knowledge, provided relief from acute disorders, and improved personal adjustment. Psychotherapy, indeed, has its place in counseling persons who are unable to adjust to society or to themselves purely on social or psychological grounds.

Pleneurethic does, however, clearly express philosophical antagonism to any form of psychotherapy that claims permanent cure of chronic illness by application of verbal bandages, conversational splints, or intellectual surgery.

PART 4

The salient ideas which distinguish the healing aspect of Pleneurethic from all other branches of the healing arts are its concept of brain sufficiency, its unlimited scope, its analytic approach, and its therapeutic techniques. Freedom from cerebellar assault provides a sense of perfect security, well-being, serenity, and mental and physical competence.

Definitive Terminology

Pleneurethic (PNE) postulates that the basis for vigorous health and good life springs from sustained and enlightened comprehension of the structures essential to cerebellar competency. It is a system of thought which provides an enduring, indissoluble ethical standard with which any person may constructively and radiantly identify. Pleneurethic relates all the affairs of the life of man to his central neural system and diagnoses the ways in which the sociological and psychological body of civilization may be collectively preserved from mental and physical deficiency. Pleneurethic integrates the study of the human organism by relating the physical, intellectual, and ethical components of the human being through a comprehensive concept of brain efficiency.

Structural Pleneurethic

Structural Pleneurethic relates the special approach of Pleneurethic to diagnosis and treatment of pathological conditions which are readily recognized by trained technological observation. Brain disturbance is caused by structural stress. Such tension originates from a complexity of sources, but invariably accumulates in the brain, which transmits the results to the somatic receptors it controls. The study of the cause and effect of brain stress and disturbance is an important aspect of Pleneurethic.

The brain, when unrestricted by influences alien to its functions, and correctly structured, responds with absolute lucidity to everything imposed upon it. But when the brain becomes sodden and destructured from chronic traumatic overburden and continued undernourishment, it responds erratically and unnaturally, if indeed it responds at all.

The brain is a universal tissue capable of omniscient directional communication with both mind and body. It is vulnerable to accidents which harm the body, especially when they affect the bioductory system.

The bioductory devices, Pleneurethic's newly discovered anatomical system, are composed of discrete neural foramina, nerviducts in long bones, lateral spinal foramen, central spinal foramen, vertebral notches, soft nerve tract sheaths which connect to nerviducts in the long bones, cranial foramen, and related sectors vital to the osseous framework to which they are adventitious.

The chief duty of the bioductory system is to permit the neural organization to retain its structural integrity as the brain performs its multifarious activities. Harmful stress and tension in the bioductory system creates correlative stress and tension of pathological dimensions in the brain and throughout the organism. The pattern of stressful disorder in the bioductories, plus acute stresses introduced into the body from other vectors, determine the composite pattern of illness. *This axiom is irrefutable, and verifies the premises inherent in Pleneurethic.*

The ethic of Pleneurethic is related to the structure of the mentality, and to neurological competence. Therefore, since Pleneurethic postulates that health is derived from overall neurological competence, it follows that the ethical mentality improves chances for well-being and success in life.

All tension imposed on the brain diminishes its capability. The brain profits from the use of a normal amount of tension, but beyond this limit, the brain may suffer damage, manifested initially in injury to microstructural forms and later in macrostructural deterioration.

Once the structure of the brain has been adversely stressed, its pathological condition will produce secondary symptoms of mental distortion and organic disorder. This secondary condition undermines the immediate environment of the brain still further, and establishes a declivitous biological trend of progressively lower levels of health, accompanied by concomitantly induced deterioration.

Pleneurethic does not classify sickness in terms of diseases.

Instead, Pleneurethic diagnoses ill health in terms of the prime cause of reduced level of brain capability. Pleneurethic does this because such diagnosis is the only reliable sign that points directly to the correct route for effective therapeutic administration.

The Pleneurethical Mind

The Pleneurethical mind is more than a quantity of intellectual power; it implies a wisdom that confers quality of thought as well. The quality of intellectual mind will be determined by the excellence of its structure. The Pleneurethic mind is not malicious, nor does it strive to belittle or overcome convictions which contribute to the peace of another person. It strives vigorously to test theories, impeach irrelevancy of principle, and joust with conniving institutions, but the Pleneurethical mind will never trifle with the psychological sanctity of another person. Preservation of human dignity is a fundamental principle of Pleneurethic.

The Pleneurethical mind speaks honestly and frankly rather than with crude brutality. Its goal is to establish honesty and sincerity in all relationships with our fellowmen. Pleneurethic is rooted in truth instead of mystery and deception.

Pleneurethic is an intellectually stimulating system of thought, philosophy, and science. Its inner core of practicality is founded upon investigative science and demonstrable clinical effectiveness. It also includes a peripheral fringe of speculative philosophy which provides an inquisitive mind ample opportunity to roam. However, the entire system is integrated and compatible, forming a logical and workable whole. It is unchallenged as the most expansive system of thought and guide to good living ever conceived.

Pleneurethic is better in its effect, and it is more rational than other systems dealing separately with mind, ethic, and chronic illness. Pleneurethic actually cures as it reverses the cause of chronic neurological tension and the resulting chronic illness process; it relieves acute psychological tension of brain tissue by restructuring mind on a proper and rational basis, and instills practical, self-responsible ethic along with natural mind development and character improvement.

Absolute Ethic

Absolute ethic is a phrase developed by Pleneurethic and is established on a belief in conduct which enhances the preservation and proper evolution of our species, as well as appropriate cultivation of the entire living community. Pleneurethic does not attempt to dictate an ethical design for any particular individual, but feels that each man is competent to evolve his own system. Pleneurethic is advantageous in that it instructs people to think humanely, and imposes individual responsibility on each person. Everyone who disciplines himself will discover the mosaic consciousness which will be verified for him through valid conceptual meanings.

The Pleneurethic attitude exhibits malice toward none and benevolence for all. Optimum freedom is guaranteed for each individual, restricted only by that which is injurious to oneself or which invades the freedom of others to live their lives without unwarranted molestation. Pleneurethic advocates an absolute rule of good conduct that will result in optimum neural sufficiency and esprit de corps both for the individual and our species en masse.

Pleneurethic prefers to be completely realistic and use an internal source of ultimate authority and responsibility for ethic. Pleneurethic is empirical, teaching people to think humanely from the morality of ethical experience, compelling them to rely on the results. A person is ultimately responsible for his conduct through his exercise of free will. Utilization of an inner source of good ethic merely squares with the living facts.

The best basis for a guiding ethic is achieved by developing our inner source of ethical power, moral insight, and universal comprehension of social circumstance. A full realization of the real worth of ourselves and others about us is achieved if we sincerely endeavor to develop personal ethical insight. Only then will we have the ethical sensitivity and comprehension to respond effortlessly in a completely moral manner in our relationship with all things in our emotional and mental environment.

Pleneurethic does not claim to have special merit as a healing profession because of superior educational collateral. Nor will Pleneurethic claim to have better, more intelligent, more dedicated men than those devoted to other therapeutic methods. However, Pleneurethic can provide more effective analysis and enduring therapy which will restore health to chronically ill persons.

Pleneurethic will not lend itself to defrauding the public by recommending or prescribing any useless product. Pleneurethic will not depart from its basic structural course of treatment of chronic illness, through reassertion of brain integrity, fidelity, and dominance by appropriate corrective methods. Pleneurethic is the key to neural control, health, and emotional stability; it illuminates the way to a more meaningful life. It is self-revealing, self-instructive, and the perfect mental science.

[Part 4 was prepared by Mr. Robert W. Shields at the author's request. He based his discussion on the original eight-volume work by R. B. Collier.]

PART 5

What is Man? What is Life?

Life on earth is an involvement of mind in flesh through brain; life is enriched as this involvement is perfected.

If flesh is denied or ethical mind abandoned or brain tissue abused, life will be distorted and ugly and unrewarding.

If flesh is acknowledged and the reach of ethical mind is honored and brain respected, life will come to have meaning beautiful to all.

Life on earth has meaning relative to the earth itself because our physical body is fashioned from the earth at hand. If the earth is poor and exhausted and corrupted, the meaning of life will tend to become deficient and restricted and distorted. Neighbor will turn against neighbor, and man will rebel within himself. If the land is rich and fertile and properly maintained, life will have all essential prerequisites for material excellence.

Life also has meaning in relation to other life. If our relationship with other life is unethical, this dereliction will impair civilization in general, deny the guilty individual full stature, and deprive his life of fullest meaning.

Life also has a reality set by brain performance. Dimension and statistics of reality for any particular individual are relative to brain capability and competence. As the brain is altered by experience or mental effort or physical trauma or battery by drugs, so is the framework of reality shifted for the mind of that particular individual.

The deepest meaning of life is not to be found in a mechanical brain; it is deeper in the nature of ma.ı. However, if mechanical brain is impaired, the inner nature of pure man will be unable to determine the true nature of the surrounding world, and it will also be unable to find faithful expression easily and effortlessly.

The destructured brain deceives the mind and punishes the body. There is no end to such torment until death terminates the process, or the brain is restructured to normal by Pleneurethical measures and the path of malady reversed.

CONCLUSION

PART 1

The professional healing picture in most of the Western world is frozen dead center by its devotion to the germ-drug theory of healing.

As a result, the largest branch of the healing profession is so hopelessly married to the commercial drug industry and the concept of germs that it cannot be salvaged by its own effort. Most of its practitioners have ceased to be real doctors of healing and have become a classy form of regular chemical salesmen earning undeserved prestige and profit through the constant support and sales efforts of the pharmaceutical industry.

It is repugnant to the public interest that powerful lobbyists of commercial chemical medicine should be able to restrain free trade in competitive healing methods and ideas. Until the advent of acupuncture they had successfully stopped ideas from permeating from the different branches of the healing sciences to the practicing physician by building up walls of prejudice and contempt. Healing based solely on the use of chemicals can be dangerous in the extreme. The pharmaceutical industry as a whole thrives under conditions that are not allowed to exist in any other industry. For instance, surface transportation interests were never permitted to suppress air travel, neither were cable communication circles permitted to stifle the transmission of messages through radio and satellite links.

That such a monopoly can be maintained by an industry in an area which concerns itself with the fitness and well-being of individuals verges on the horrific.

Drug medicine is not perfect. Neither is psychiatry, osteopathy, chiropractic, naturopathy, acupuncture or Japanese Finger

Pressure. But out of the mistakes made by each a more perfect system of healing can be evolved. Pleneurethic itself could not have evolved without the mistakes of other drug and nondrug oriented schools of thought.

It is unrealistic, even fraudulent, to consire to restrain competition among the various healing groups. Developmental errors are sometimes made, but an occasional mistake or series of them should not be enough to stifle a project, especially when no other project in the same general field has been completely successful.

It is interesting to note that after I published a work outlining the concept of Pleneurethic a major medical discovery was reported by a popular magazine. It was that millions of children had been needlessly placed in mental institutions because their condition had been maldiagnosed. It was found that their basic problem was physical and not mental. Worse, the "new diagnosis" was based on alleged research carried out shortly after World War II which had been "lost" for close to thirty years.

The article said many of the affected children had minimal brain damage. This is another way of saying that they suffered from neural insufficiency, but that term is not as accurate because it overlooks the peripheral neural system, which is in the spinal cord, and the bioductory system. Interestingly, many of the children were injured at birth. We should note in passing that minimal brain damage will not respond properly to a biochemical communication, surgery, or psychotherapy. Therefore, healing progress cannot be made with these unfortunate children until physical correction of their bioductory disorder has been inaugurated.

Unfortunately, no person has as yet been taught by the author to practice healing by the Pleneurethic method, but when a few are taught their number will grow; and, because they will be encouraged to seek and think and expand on ideas, their ultimate contribution to medicine and mankind will be great.

The need for them was strikingly illustrated by a prominent American pediatrician who recently announced that he had made a breakthrough in the treatment of children with behavioral and learning problems. He realized that these children did not have the deep psychological problems that other professionals had long thought to be the main cause of their condition. Instead, he said, they were suffering from brain traumas often so slight that they could not be measured by conventional devices.

The pediatrician was reported to be experimenting with drugs to treat the condition. He was acting on the assumption that as the small child was hyperexcited and could not concentrate he could best be helped by being given a drug which would excite his ability to reject distracting noises.

But, according to the article, treatment with depressant drugs did not produce the desired results, and the children were then given drugs to raise their level of excitement.

No doubt many of the children are hyperexcited, cannot concentrate, and have behavioral problems because they possess bioductory system trauma arising from inept obstetrics or a fall from the crib. They need biomechanical correction to stabilize and relax their chronically excited brains—not to have their already much abused delicate neurological system further abused by biochemical stimulants. Unfortunately, I feel that the self-seeking pharmaceutical scourge will not be terminated until training in medical colleges is aligned more closely to coincide with my Pleneurethical views on the diagnosis and treatment of chronic illness.

PART 2

In this age of cynicism and disillusionment, man more than ever before needs to believe in something above himself, but which is still of this world. This need is best placed in the goodness of civilization or the progress of humankind. In the pressures that surround us today man has tended to forget that no man is entirely self-sufficient. To have a full life he must rely upon other people. The recognition of this need will go a long way toward creating a true aura of neighborly love throughout the world.

With this in mind, Pleneurethic aims its program for the improvement of civilization at people and not at institutions.

For, as people uplift their ethical comprehension, errant institutions will spontaneously flex into proper alignment with the flow of new times.

Therefore, the restructuring of social abuse should not include a program designed specifically to destroy unacceptable institutions. This would accomplish nothing. Rather, it would leave the way open for the establishment of a new institutional order which may easily be more off center than the one that was destroyed. Institutions are improper simply because they reflect the impropriety of the people at large.

Pleneurethic encourages individual men and women, who constitute civilization, to garb themselves in better ethical raiment. Once they have improved their ethical posture, the structure of institutions will shift effortlessly in sympathy with the new structure of civilization.

Pleneurethic envisages a new civilization. In it armies will still be maintained, but their mission will be mercy, not mayhem. Their job will be to combat natural disasters and build defenses against nature's occasional and brutal offensives.

A ministry of ethic will carry the scepter of ethic to men, women, and children in the world so they may refine their own inner temple of moral nobility.

There will be schools, but practice will come along with theory. The hospitals, the homes for the aged, the bakeries, the farms, the mines, the foundries, the factories, and the financial institutions will be extensions of the classrooms.

Teachers will be working people who are competent to teach the art of their trade, the principles of their trade, and the knowledge required to successfully carry out their trade or profession.

Instead of competing in exams, students will work together in teams and the teams will be set projects which will be of continuing benefit to civilization. Students will rotate among the teams as they progress through the curriculum of the school. There will be no graduation, and the student will be able to drop out to assume a position in society or reenter the education system at will, whenever he or she wishes to continue training.

By serving the real needs of society the individual best serves himself or herself and the people about him or her.

Civilization can be ruined in many ways. It can be ruined through the unbridled reign of exuberant but inexperienced youth or, conversely, through the complete dominance of sternly inflexible elders. Civilization can also be spoiled through man's inability to understand himself and his environment.

This is why Pleneurethic endeavors to build an improved civilization by helping each person to understand things and the people about him in terms of cerebellar economy.

The Pleneurethical person understands the desperate problem of youth, whose robust neural system confers a natural feeling of exquisite competency and invincibility, yet whose inexperience of mind and skinny seed of real wisdom can easily lead him astray.

The tragedy of youth lies in the extensive mismatch between the neurological capability of his brain and the experienced knowledge of his mind. Because of this, youth does not know that the lack of practical experience in the mature affairs of adult life leaves it shallowly unfit for the role fleet and burgeoning neural energies mislead it to believe it is fully qualified for. Therefore, youth is unable to know that premature demands are solid evidence of immaturity and signs of a person who has not yet prepared himself for leadership.

Youth must be taught to look to elders for lessons of eternal wisdom pried loose by these voyages of the past from nature's storehouse of knowledge. If youth does not do so, and is forced to acquire experience and knowledge through his own errors, another discrepancy develops. That is that the youth suddenly finds his neurological capability shorter than his knowledge. Almost without knowing it he has grown old and shaky and sometimes socially bad tempered. His potential for advancing civilization is virtually lost.

Therefore, the duties of youth and age are to understand each other. Youth and age are interdependent and have to work closely and patiently together if they are to form a really fruitful and progressive civilization, a civilization which forges surely ahead as more refined thought and action replaces that which has become outmoded, impractical, or injurious.

Youth and age must learn to understand both strengths and weaknesses of each other's position in the stream of civilization's evolution. As it is, young people sincerely search for the good and the true but they are exploited at nearly every turn. From childhood, youth is bombarded with masses of misleading information extensively publicized as facts of truth by special interest groups. Much of this "brain-washing" mentality warping nonsense, masquerading as fact, is cleverly introduced bit by bit into children's textbooks and by youthful teachers themselves who were similarly conditioned. This is why I believe no teacher should be allowed to teach until he or she has spent ten years earning his or her own living outside the schoolroom.

Many young people are now handicapped and forestalled from perceiving the true because they already believe intuitively and implicitly in certain popular doctrines which are in fact fallacious in pure structured science. Others, in desperation, turn to far-out philosophies and strange practices seeking answers they have been denied by self-occupied elders who more often than not are inclined to perpetuate and magnify past mistakes in civilization.

To introduce a brand new philosophy rooted in pure science is difficult enough, but to overcome the inertia of powerful pre-existing institutions grown fat and ugly by milking the people is nearly impossible.

Pleneurethic starts from a basic point, which is simple enough. Yet in the detail of its application the system grows complicated at an ever-accelerating rate.

Yet this should not be so strange. Nature uses this method. For example, take the sun. The notion that the sun is important to the people in the world is simple. It just rests there in the heavens and shines. But when we commence seeing how the sun causes moisture to rise from the waters of the earth, sometimes in the form of fog and sometimes in invisible form, plants to grow, marked changes in the habits of animal movements, winter and summer, the subject grows more complicated.

So it is with Pleneurethic.

It commences from the notion that a very important thing in life, perhaps the single most important thing, is the brain, its structure and energy.

Once the notion is applied it becomes exceptionally complicated very quickly. Especially as it has an impact in such divergent fields as philosophy, psychology, religion, and healing. As such it fosters the grasp of truth, reality, and ethic.

At this twentieth-century juncture, cerebellar strengths and weaknesses are least well understood, and most often grossly misunderstood, by lay and professionals alike. That this is true will become apparent if institutions of civilizations are examined from the standpoint of neural economy. Many world institutions—particularly in the fields of religion, psychology, medicine, and government—are vulnerable to indictment for failure to properly consider the neural system individually and collectively and its limitations. Some schools of mystical philosophy advocating the use of exotic drugs to unnaturally expand the mind may actually harm brain tissue. Such drugs, therefore, have little real value as a way of life in Pleneurethic.

Central neural competency is man's most basic value. With this enlightened resource all things of this world are available to the possessor. Without it nothing is available, not even the strength to breathe the ubiquitous air, or the stamina to develop wisdom or beauty or grace. Without it a man becomes a burden on civilization rather than one who supports it and enhances its potential for advancement.

Values achieve significance and universal acceptance because of their usefulness. Almost everything in the world, seen and unseen, has some amount of usefulness in one way or another. Some things have much more usefulness than others and are coveted when their supply is limited.

In Pleneurethic it is postulated that the most useful thing is sufficient cerebellar capability. Without this vital resource vigor of thought itself is curtailed, along with a reduction of physical competency. The length of life is also governed by the state of neurological competency.

Brain furnishes the power for life, and to function properly it requires proper management. Good brain management requires a host of things ranging from the structure of our mentality and the food we eat to the way we exert ourselves physically and mentally and the accidents we permit our bodies to suffer.

The most essential thing to a long and good life is the satisfactory set of the bioductory system. If this can be maintained throughout one's life, the brain and its extensions will always enjoy a hospitable earthly abode. The brain will manifest a condition interpreted by the mind as great well-being. The body will seem indestructible and nondegradable. The fortunate possessor will luxuriate in a long and good life.

If, on the other hand, the bioductory system is damaged, the brain will begin to steadily deteriorate and death will come earlier than if the system were maintained in good health. As well as having a diminished life expectancy, the person with a damaged bioductory system will feel in his mind that his body is suffering discomfort. He will also experience actual physical disease and will suffer chronic mental upsets, which will give him a tendency to behave abnormally at times.

PART 3

In Pleneurethic there is a program for optimum health and endurance which contains a number of basic elements. It applies to the balance and stamina of the mind as well as to the body. If the brain is properly cared for, the body and mentality will have an enduring bulwark on which it can confidently rely and the transition period leading to death, when it comes, will be peaceful.

The program for health includes things to avoid and things to be done. A number of things are to be avoided if we are to retain the optimum level of brain performance. To determine them one general rule is to avoid all things that injure the brain either directly or indirectly. Light irritations over a long period of time will damage brain capability just as surely as heavier trauma over a shorter period. Moreover, those things which injure the brain may seem unimportant and irrelevant to the person who is not knowledgeable in this new field of thought. This is evidenced by some of the case histories discussed earlier.

Serious injury to the very complicated casing system (the bioductory system) that surrounds and protects the central neural system must be avoided. Serious injury can come from falling from a highchair, a tree, or a horse. Careless and ill-considered use of obstetric instruments can cause serious damage as can misadventures on a sports field. Heavy twisting or bending or lifting, as in golf and housework, when it is incorrectly done can also lead to serious trouble.

Excessive alcohol consumption, drug addiction, and many medicines provide sure routes to brain deterioration and early death, to say nothing of irreversible damage to the brains of fetuses in expectant mothers who take alcohol and other poisons in excessive quantities.

Excessive food or improper food can also take its toll over the years. Malnutrition in prenatal or infant stages may irreversibly damage brain capability and development.

Excessive acquisition of useless knowledge can overload the brain and contribute to reduced efficiency.

Any assault to the senses should be avoided. Excessive noise from heavy traffic, airports or construction sites can cause damage. So can loud music from powerful electronic amplifiers. All of these can damage the brain's capability before destroying the auditory apparatus and nullifying it as an avenue through which damaging stress may be transmitted to the brain.

Heated arguments and anger seriously overload the brain and are capable of causing illness in a young person and death in an elderly person.

Unsolved problems should be solved as soon as possible because they encumber substantial resources of brain capability unproductively.

Excessive social life can also place an excessive and debilitating load on the brain, and so can the embarkation on too many projects. Therefore, it is better to concentrate one's effort in relatively few directions.

If we have offended anyone it is better to seek immediate forgiveness, or otherwise redress ourselves, than to permit ourselves to wallow in mental anguish which will continue to assault our neural reserves.

However, of all of the things to avoid the most significant is injury to the bioductory system. The seriousness of such injury overshadows all else. Such things as loud noises or unsolved problems are not likely in themselves to cause chronic mental illness, but they may reinforce chronic stresses already installed in the brain through bioductory tension and contribute to mental and physical collapse from overall neurological exhaustion.

Death which follows brain failure is usually and erroneously diagnosed as heart attack by medical authority. [Please refer to volume 1 of *Pleneurethic,* published in early 1965, for further information on this subject.]

What can be done to produce health?

First of all the paramount significance of the brain must be recognized and life must be ordered in keeping with the capabilities and limitation of the brain.

We must lead moderate lives except in the areas in which we wish to excel. Even there, we must be careful not to overtax ourselves in the short term because that will impede performance in the long term.

Good character, derived from ethical development plus moderate physical exercise along with adequate diet, sufficient rest, and honorable work, will go a long way toward creating health.

Injuries to the bioductory system caused through accidents or heavy exertion can often be reversed by Pleneurethical biomechanical methods. But at present there are no schools in operation to produce doctors trained in these methods and, therefore, one has to be doubly wary of all circumstances which in a split second can cause injury which may ruin bioductory system health and blight the remaining period of life.

Pleneurethic then, in stark summary, envisions a rational basis for life, and advocates the personal acceptance of each individual's own responsibility for shaping his or her own destiny. It teaches a system of health and morality that is impartially applicable to all peoples and all parts of the globe. The teaching focuses upon constructive economy of man's neurological resources. The approach is structural, because from a study of structure springs a clear perception of truth.

Pleneurethic is predicated upon structure, which gives it an indestructible basis in truth and logic. Its final goal is to elevate civilization through the raising of each person's ethical character and constructive productivity, so that all people will be able to live in harmony with themselves and their environment.

APPENDIX 1

Mr. Moderator, members of the panel, ladies and gentlemen: Thank you all for being here. I wish to give special thanks to the directors of Interim 1977 for allowing Pleneurethic to be a part of their program at Whitman College, and to the members of this panel for consenting to appear. They possess many enviable abilities, paramount among them is the facility for translating my cumbersome and tedious Pleneurethical writing into language currently in use on campus, hence more readily accessible to students. Now to the business of this moment, which is to examine some Pleneurethical philosophy, and its extension which forms a new science and way of life.

Philosophy means different things to different people. In Pleneurethic it refers to the basic reason for doing a thing. It is a guiding principle for disciplined thought and action.

Some philosophies are relatively narrow in their field of application. They are ideologues, and often conflict with other equally narrow philosophies which strike them full force or encroach tangentially. The result is confusion among the people about the basic realities of life. They have difficulty in solving fundamental life problems satisfactorily. Arguments occur and strife is rampant. Living energy, that could better be devoted to improving personal health or to uplifting the quality of life in our civilization, is wasted.

Pleneurethic outlines a philosophy which is universal in scope, and hence has the potential for integrating virtually the total spectrum of human behavior. Pleneurethic establishes a clear

This appendix is the edited version of a speech delivered by the author at Whitman College, Walla Walla, Washington, on January 7, 1977.

interdisciplinary target which effectively points us toward meaningful curricular reform in colleges, with possible onward benefit to our nation.

The practice of Pleneurethic, in fostering the basis for health in our world community, is predicated upon a new structural science which is inherent in the unique philosophy of Pleneurethic. The professional practice of Pleneurethic involves difficult and dangerous techniques which are best discussed and demonstrated in the disciplined atmosphere of a university classroom, attended by qualified persons seeking professional status in the new field of Pleneurethic.

The techniques are difficult, in part, because of subtle complexities in the mentality and the bioductory system, and the infinite variety of ways in which they deteriorate under inimical stresses generated by structural derangements. The techniques of bioductory rehabilitation are potentially dangerous because physical restructuring forces, if misapplied by impetuous and unskilled operators, may intensify rather than attenuate or reverse the chronic illness process. The practice of the science of Pleneurethic deals with the brain and the several surrounding environments which impact upon the macrostructure and microstructure of brain to alter its function. This is an immensely difficult and vast body of knowledge for the student to master. Any mistakes made by the therapist, in diagnosis or execution or application of physical or psychic restructuring forces, create hardship or death to the patient because of the paramount significance of the brain in the health and disease process.

Philosophy is always a serious matter and leads to serious debate. For example, two college debaters testing their mettle over such subjects as evolution or immaculate conception. However, once the debate is concluded, each participant continues life relatively unscathed. This is not true of more serious controversy centered on the correct philosophy of healing. Here the debate affects the dying patient and the person who presumes to act as doctor. If the philosophy is wrong, the science and practice which emerge from the philosophy are ineffective or even detrimental. The patient departs to an early grave, and the physician, depressed by the needless death, finds little ground for jubilation in the fact that he himself remains alive to collect the bill for unsuccessful services rendered.

Lay people and professionals alike must understand *why* things are done if they are to comprehend the basis for achievement of a consistently proper course of action. The *why* of doing a thing is actually the *principle* or philosophy upon which that action is based. Principles, then, are important to us because they form a solid and enduring basis for effective performance. They provide a reason and logic for our thinking, and permit a continuity to activity. They allow critical evaluation of the merit of our guiding knowledge.

Principles, at play in the world, come in layers. Some are pretty much on the surface and are easily apparent. But, behind the obvious exterior layer resides another layer, and behind this other layers until we eventually come to the First Cause—the Prime Principle, the Absolute Principle. Somewhere along the line of interconnecting principle, we commence to name it philosophy or theology—depending upon our calling and on our ability to reason rationally. This philosophy, principle, or reason why, is applied to all action which is reasonable and accountable in an educated and enlightened culture.

Philosophy is especially important in healing, and the thoughtful physician who would save himself and his profession from charges of ineptitude or downright charlatanry, must be a philosopher as well as a practicing healer. And his philosophy must be joined with a consuming love for truth and logic, rather than expediency and a desire for fiscal prominence along with a lavish display of wealth and opulence around the community. For surely it is so, the physician who is captured by a wish for a high life style and social prominence and financial wealth may never be a true healer.

The physician who is not also a philosopher is severely limited by his training. He can do only that which he is trained to do. He dare not deviate, for he has no philosophy to guide him, nor is he able to devise new treatments to meet novel situations. He lacks the unerringly accurate flexibility of a philosopher. Most assuredly he cannot successfully challenge therapy based upon superstition and maudlin myth or commercial chicanery. The clinician takes pride in his training; the heavily practicing physician points to his school and his license. But the genuine philosopher, the master working philosopher—and there have been precious few—takes some small offense when asked where he gained his knowledge and who trained him and what entity of government licensed him or why is he not licensed.

The master working philosopher travels in uncharted and sometimes hazardous regions. He creates insight where there was none before, and must attempt to construe new notions and theoretical bases for novel practices; otherwise he is not such a philosopher. The master working philosopher labors unceasingly to create the ability of thinking for himself in unmarked regions of knowledge, takes responsibility for his own inner refinement, and demands strict ethical accountability of himself for all his decisions and actions. Such personal development is not easily achieved, nor is it easily maintained once acquired. It is accomplished only after decades of grueling effort. It is helpful if such serious effort is commenced early in life.

People of Pleneurethic should encourage their children, commencing at a very early age to be self-reliant, take responsibility for the consequences of their decisions and actions, and live according to ethical principles. For unless this is accomplished by parents or guardians, children may not discover it by themselves or recognize the importance of such inner refinement until too late. Some, regrettably, may never realize it.

Indeed, the grand work of life, according to *Pleneurethic,* volume 3, published in 1967, is to develop the inner resources to reflect ethical principles in all things. The paramount decision in the Pleneurethical way of life is to personally choose the ethical way over the careless way, and to dedicate one's energy to searching out and embracing eternal ethical principles.

The following must be underscored in bold: Pleneurethical people do not follow the ethical life, they forge it. The ethical way may not always be the easy way to perceive or to negotiate. Quite to the contrary, the ethical way is often a very difficult way, especially in the beginning. We, individually, must clear away the massive boulders of self-service and prickly scrub brush of deceit which obscure our ethical path. Such work may be exceptionally difficult, but no real progress is made toward self-mastery until it is commenced in unmitigated earnestness. And there are other impediments beside boulders and scrub brush which must be tended, but enumerating them would belabor the point.

If we faithfully await for some god to effortlessly endow us with eternal ethical illumination, we may languish in vain. The Absolute of Pleneurethic is not conceived to operate in such fashion. The Absolute simply furnishes the tools. We must learn through arduous practice to employ them skillfully, thereby uplifting the level of civilization and enhancing our own unselfish portion of it.

The concept of the Absolute is necessary to our study of Pleneurethical affairs because Pleneurethic considers all of the various environments which impact upon the several brains of humankind. In a way, Pleneurethic's concept of the Absolute is the most important environment of all. Perhaps it should have been the leading chapter in my latest book—*Pleneurethic and the Brain*—because of its pervasive and compelling influence upon the cultural institutions of civilization, and also because of the great mischief which may be imposed upon humankind by the way in which theologians and ministers of the numerous Gospels extant conceive the First Cause to be structured. Once these temporal architects of church have structured their special God to their spiritual satisfaction, the gentle people of the flock are expected to conform to the dictates of rigid ecclesiastical canon. Sometimes great strain is shoveled by clerics upon people, this by virtue of the agonizing discontinuity between unrealistic and overly stern church requirements and human capability and credulity.

Pleneurethic considers the total person; therefore, we cannot avoid evaluation of the religious environment which influences that person. Actually, the religious environment is a part of the social or cultural environment, but with a peculiar pathological convolution. Many religionists declare that people are nothing but spirit, and they are healthy or disease-ridden simply because of that spirit. These religionists, theologians, and practicing ministers declare that the cure for all illness is through control of the Holy Spirit exclusively. Hence, prayers, blessings, exorcisms, and the like, are the only ways these churchmen seek to treat all manner of diseases. They deny the effectiveness of chemical or physical or psychic restructuring by temporal physicians. Since the Holy Spirit is said by some theologians to be an essence of God—the First Cause of the universe and all that is in it—we cannot avoid a critical discussion of such matters if we are to understand Pleneurethic philosophy, which underpins the proper treatment of the composite person by way of cerebellar rehabilitation. Volume 3 of *Pleneurethic* went into a lengthy discussion of the characteristics of God, and the Absolute. Hence, the discussion of the book entitled *Pleneurethic and the Brain* was of necessity summary and cursory only.

Pleneurethic bases its philosophy upon structure. It recognizes a harmonious compatibility among the physical structure of man, the physical structure of the universe, and the structural essence of the Absolute—First Cause—or *Pleneurethical God*. Indeed, the Absolute of Pleneurethic is the central structure from whose zenith all other structures and substructures of this world and this universe devolve. Moreover, the *spiritual philosophy of Pleneurethic* involves nothing but a study of the unseen structures which reside behind the physics of worldly structures as seen by our eyes, felt with our fingers, heard with our ears, and palpated by cerebellar acquity along with a sympathetic mentality.

The compatibility, between the physics courses in your local college and the metaphysics of Pleneurethic, is virtually total. Therefore, the metaphysical philosophy of Pleneurethic is not some nebulous flight of self-serving denominational imagination, but rather it is a firm, down-to-earth, disciplined extrapolation of the characteristics of our physical universe.

Self-care and self-responsibility versus submission to an

external patron institution who ministers each person's needs: this basic choice in life has plagued people since the beginning. It pervades all affairs of humankind.

We see it in religion and church, whereby the people are expected to relinquish responsibility for their lives and become humble sheep tended by an authoritative shepherd in starched ministerial collar. We see it in government, when the people are exhorted to look up to lofty government for fulfillment of all needs, rather than to care for themselves through their own industry. We also see it in healing, when the people are kept ignorant of true healing techniques by commercial drug medicine and in subsequent ill health are schooled to seek help solely in the neighborhood pharmacy and in the nearby clinic exclusively.

Unfortunately, there is at present a difference between pure science and modern medicine. The one is dedicated to unselfishly searching out the truth, the other all too often to fiscal exploitation of people through the avenue of pharmacy. Now science, just this year, has recognized and stated publicly that diseases such as cancer and heart attack are not "caught" like a cold is allegedly "caught," but result from years of thoughtless abuse to the body, and that miracle drugs will not heal such diseases. To put the record straight, out of all fairness, I must stipulate: some medical doctors are also scientists. However, they seem to be in the minority. Moreover, they are unpardonably tardy in their recognition of proper health principles.

In 1963 Pleneurethic was conceived by me (it was published in printed form in 1964); its basic message was health and the good life through an understanding of eternal health principles— *Pleneurethical principles.* These principles, based on a pure structural science of the brain and its several environments, were at variance with what was at that time being circulated by orthodox healing interests in the medical colleges, and demanded as answers to questions by state licensing bureaus. Among other things, these Pleneurethical principles stressed the notion that if people could understsand the true nature of their being and live accordingly, their chances for disease-free life could be enhanced.

The prime tenet of Pleneurethic philosophy, then, is that

people must take responsibility for their own affairs, including their own health, insofar as possible. Self-care is based upon true knowledge of *Pleneurethical reality* and how one's body, brain, and mind really work, and upon what the universe really is, and the person's proper relationship with the laws which provide the matrix within which both man and the universe must operate.

Of course, Pleneurethic does not advocate self-care in all things. But it does recommend that people in general, homemakers in particular, and children wherever possible, be encouraged to study Pleneurethic principles and science and practice. If they will do this, and become reasonably knowledgeable in this new field of ethic and health, they will increase chances for a productive, disease-free life. People should realize they are not free to diminish the structure of their brain through habitual maleating, hateful abuse of others, intemperate use of drugs and alcohol, unbridled sensuality, or bioductory-rending athletics. Such abuse to their person is unethical because of its negative impact upon themselves and a struggling world civilization.

Children should be taught to guard their future health by prudent living, from day to day, in a manner calculated to preserve brain competence. They should be taught to recognize and avoid dangerous living practices. They should be instructed that, despite their virtually inexhaustible bounce-back energy and apparent invulnerability to harmful things, these things are treacherous and accumulate over the years to attenuate cerebellar capability and to increase vulnerability to all sorts of mental and physical and emotional diseases later on in life. Some of these diseases come slowly in later years with adequate warning. Others strike like a heavy storm at sea, and the person is drowned in a flash with no time to find a lifeboat or reshape his ship to weather the vicious storm. Smarter or wiser living, then, requires that students be taught bioductory mechanics in school, as well as ethical mental mechanics and good brain management. These three things profoundly influence our person and our chances for a healthy life.

To recapitulate: If we grasp Pleneurethical principles we will realize that serious chronic illnesses are not fortuitously acquired by bacterial or viral misfortune; rather, we deliberately lay the rotten foundation for these illnesses on our own negligence or careless living excesses. And the disease-prone pattern is inaugurated by people, usually in their childhood, youth, and young adulthood. Miracle drugs, no matter how potent, can never really and truly reverse the impact of an improper life-style because they are incapable of correctively restructuring gross anatomy, and they are also unable to restore chronic distortion of brain structure and capability to normal.

Once the brain commences its progressive path of pathological deterioration under the overburdening impact of accidents to the bioductory system and long-term neurological overdrafts from excessive living, the chronically diseased person does not think well, hence is unable to solve problems that could have been easily handled in earlier and healthier days. Moreover, as our brain structure deteriorates, so also does body structure and function decline, and thereby undermine the healthful environmental basis for the brain at ever-accelerating rates. We may never reach old age, and if we do, we are frequently occupants of state facilities and an unwelcome tax liability upon those who have lived more prudently.

Crowning achievement in Pleneurethical ethic is to conduct our lives in such manner that we are able to add to the upward thrust of our nation's civilization, and not detract from it or depress it for others by our own neglectful misconduct or failure to develop all our personal faculties and resources. Surely we are most ethical when we live our lives in a healthful way, and avoid those harmful things which will cause us to be disease-prone, and a burden on world society in the future.

APPENDIX 2

Spiritual Healing

PART 1

Justification for investigation of spiritual healing springs from claims by priests to competency in the cure of chronic illness, by spiritual methods, through mysterious control of the Holy Spirit.

Does the church really possess the power to manipulate the Holy Spirit, thereby enabling church to permanently lift the impress of chronic illness on people? Or is church engaged in wishful thinking? Even worse, does church utter false assertions simply to convert as many people as possible for the benefit of religious combines? Church combines are very powerful. We dare not challenge church on basic questions lightly.

More to the point, is church so spiritually sacred and secularly formidable that we dare not test it at all?

A brilliant and celebrated jurist put it succinctly, no truth is so sacred it cannot be challenged. Truth challenged will prevail, be it the truth. Be it falsehood it will fall, and justly so, to the benefit of all. Truth defended successfully is rewarding, for through the work of erecting our defense, we achieve reinvigorated perception of our cherished truth. Truth unsuccessfully defended is also rewarding, for through defeat we emerge into a new era of enlightenment.

The ethical way of healthful life and healing philosophy of Pleneurethic is based upon reality and truth. We, therefore, press forward without fear in our examination of church and its spiritual healing.

PART 2

Spiritual healing commenced thousands of years ago when little was known of anatomy, physiology, biochemistry, and the like. Whereas other modes of healing have changed drastically over the centuries as additional biological information became available, spiritual healing has not felt the need to change in the slightest.

As psychotherapists have many variations on the repressed conflict theme, and the drug people have a mind-boggling array of different germs and antidotes, so it is that there are a multitude of variations on the main theme of disease due to problems involving the Holy Spirit. There are countless ways, according to the clergy, whereby a person may offend the Holy Spirit and suffer physical disease and mental torment as a result.

When spiritual healers come forth and announce themselves to be perfectly competent to cure chronic illness, they thereby insinuate themselves into the temporal affairs of the professional field of healing. More important, when they advertise themselves not to be the last resort in healing chronic illness, but rather to be the first line of defense preceding all other professional healers, they open themselves to impartial investigation. Finally, when they proclaim themselves to be "higher" than ordinary doctors they most assuredly invite rational investigation.

Beyond our physical senses, and outside the scope of the intellectual portion of our total mentality, exists a world which is intangible only because our severely attenuated senses cannot span the total vibratory spectrum to perceive it. It is in this world beyond the range of our senses, the *metaworld,* where we will find the forces of metamaterial and metaconsciousness which make our human anatomy and our human consciousness possible.

It is to this metaworld that the spiritual healers allegedly direct their attention. It is in the metaworld that the church's alleged Holy Spirit is said to reside. All forms of spiritual healing claim to employ an alleged supernatural ingredient. This supernatural force, or Holy Spirit, is supposedly utilized in a multitude of different ways. The end result is alleged to be identical; i.e., instantaneous healing of the chronic affliction.

Manipulation of the Holy Spirit is said to be accomplished by briefly laying of sacred hands on the skull of the afflicted, affirmation of divine principle by the healer, establishing a spiritual covenant with the divine, rejecting the flesh, awakening to the Holy Spirit through sacramental observance, instilling realization that disease is unnatural and can be healed by supernatural miracle, applying the charged healing atmosphere of common worship, bestowing blessing through religious benediction, etc.

Whatever conclusion one eventually develops concerning spiritual healing, any unbiased observer is forced to admit that for sheer splendor of syntax and majesty of vocabulary the clergy have matchless superiority over all other healing professions by an uneclipsable margin.

Before going onward it is only fair to tell the reader that Pleneurethic does not advocate the existence of a Holy Spirit which has a deliberate hand in making people chronically ill. We doubt the existence of any spiritual force of this design and purpose. Moreover, we do not hold in reverence any theory about the existence of such a force, even if it is declared to exist by highest priestly authority.

It is the thesis of Pleneurethic that activity of persons in this world cannot influence the so-called Holy Spirit to cure chronic illness in themselves or others. No matter what the special training of the individual, nor how mysterious his incantations, motions, and suggestions, he cannot influence the so-called Holy Spirit in the slightest degree one way or another.

It is hoped that the author will be forgiven for not being filled with awe or swooning adoration at the mention of the Holy Spirit. He cannot sanctify nor hold in devotional awe anything which, according to the ministry, causes such extensive suffering and disease among men. He does not hold in awe the psychological theory of chronic illness due to hysterical conversion, nor is he overwhelmed by the commercial drug doctors' views on chronic illness due to germs or virus. And in the same token he is definitely not respectful of the clergyman's Holy Spirit which allegedly causes heartbreaking chronic illness and tragedy among the innocent mortals of this world.

PART 3

It is an exceptional person who refuses to agree that there is not some Absolute source of universal power which either established the universe as we see, feel, and hear it, or provided for our human ability to perceive and speculate on the universe. Nearly all persons wish to assume the existence of an Absolute. However, we all disagree as to the exact properties of such an Absolute source of all force, unless, of course, we have accepted our ideas blindly as a package along with some regular religion adopted in the past.

Concepts of ultimate power in the universe have been discussed both by theologians and philosophers. Whereas theologians are preoccupied with a more or less specific concept of ultimate power because of their church ties, *philosophers* have no such connection and *are inclined to be more tolerant in the face of disagreement*. Moreover, philosophers are inclined to consider a wider range of possibilities than theologians, who insist stoutly upon a narrow concept which will support: their church, their dogma, and a vast array of spiritual offices for incumbency by major and minor church officials and priests.

If you disagree with a theologian and his followers they may kill you. This has happened in the past on a grand scale and no doubt will happen in the future. No such problem occurs with philosophers and their followers.

The various concepts of the ultimate principle have been formulated by theologians and speculative philosophers and given names such as theism.

The term *theism* is used to refer to the idea of a God of superhuman characteristics. Monotheism implies the existence of but one God, and polytheism then refers to a system of many such gods. The theistic God is the source of all existence, is separate from the universe, but is available on a personal basis with people.

Theism is not a religion but is a speculative theory which forms a core around which a religion may be constructed. If the speculative theory is shown to be false, the church and its religion is without basis, and all priests and officials of that religion and church will be without a means of livelihood. They may be expected to argue heatedly for their cause.

Positive correlation between belief in theism and good health cannot be established, nor is there any predictable relationship between disbelief in a theistic God and chronic illness. Some of the healthiest people of the world are agnostics. And if one travels extensively about the world, entire nations are to be discovered where the people are absolutely atheistic, yet their inhabitants are the very picture of health.

Animals, fishes, and birds are quite healthy but have not the capability for fine speculation on theistic matters. Indeed, good health does not directly derive from any particular intellectual concept of the origin of the universe.

I am interested only in that which really, truly, and invariably leads to a cure of the chronically ill mind and body. All alleged cures are to be regarded unemotionally and dispassionately until evidence mounts to enable decision regarding their efficacy. It is in this impartial light that we must assess the merit of the Holy Spirit in its alleged role of controller of health and illness on earth.

To Pleneurethic, the Holy Spirit of the clergyman is no more sacred than the germ theory to the pharmacists, the psychological repression theory to the psychotherapists, or the colonic irrigation to the advocate of physical therapy. They are all, including the clergy, engaged in the commerce of attempting to earn a livelihood by advertising themselves to be competent to heal all illnesses.

From the standpoint of the public welfare, if the Holy Spirit cannot be used effectively and predictably by all clergymen equally, to heal chronic illness, then the system is to be denounced as simply another racket whose only value is to produce a living for its proponents.

Some spiritual healers lay it down, "For an eye to be blind, a leg to be paralyzed, a lung to be eaten up with tuberculosis, and for a mind to be clouded with fear—these are the unnatural things." Such unnatural things can be healed according to spiritual healing philosophy with "perfect understanding and command of God and the Holy Spirit."

I do not hesitate to admit that *if* such ailments as those noted above are indeed unnatural, they then are not of this world but of another. Such things then are unnatural, oddly mysterious, and without question require knowledge in diagnosis and treatment beyond the capability of any mortal man.

Destruction of the entire array of spiritual healing apology predicated on the inherent unnaturalness of chronic disease is accomplished quite easily. The fatal mistake occurs in the major premise which dogmatizes chronic somatic illness such as blindness, paralysis, tuberculosis, and cloudy mind to be examples of *unnatural* things. In reality, things are to be classed as unnatural only if the cause is not known, and are classed as natural if the cause is known.

Pleneurethic knows the cause of such examples of disease as the chronic illnesses listed above. The cause is not in the realm of mystery, requiring an alleged spiritual healing application of supernatural power. Rather, the cause is in the temporal realm and requires application of restructuring physical force on the traumatized bioductory system to restore the brain and neural system to normal operational capability and balance.

We are not scoffing at spiritual healers, for their breach of wisdom is understandable. Their theories were developed thousands of years before Christ and perfected during the early Christian era. During these periods little was known of anatomy, and the physiology of the chronic illness process. It was, therefore, easy for early thinkers to mistake the real cause of chronic illness and consider it to be of unnatural and mysterious genesis. Moreover, they mistook the sudden but temporary release of energy based upon faith to be a cure when in fact it was only palliative.

It is equally natural and nonmysterious for a body to have arthritis, cancer, or tuberculosis if the bioductory system and brain are damaged, as it is for a bird to be grounded because of a fractured wing, or chewing to be impossible because of broken teeth. No amount of prayer will, in itself and alone, set and mend a broken wing or fix broken teeth. Nor will prayer or extreme spiritual insight by itself reposture a bioductory system chronically damaged or disordered through physical trauma.

Chronic illness is not unnatural, even though it is unwanted, despised, and not understood by the sufferer or the clergy. Chronic illness is simply a syndrome of physical, chemical, and mental symptoms which occur through operation of the natural adaptative forces built into a living body to compensate as best it can after trauma has disturbed its original and natural integrity.

And these adaptations result in such things as calciferous depositions and solidifications along a traumatized bioductory system, neural insufficiencies, organic malfunction, muscle debility, joint immobility, cancer cell development due to alterations in body chemistry, vague but intense feelings of guilt, an anxious mind, etc. All this and much more occurs when internal bioductory disorders are destroying the brain and neural system, upsetting biochemical balances, and corrupting all body functions directly or indirectly.

All such somatic adaptations and mental upsets as the preceding seem exceptionally mysterious and incomprehensible to the priestly opportunist who does not understand, does not care to understand, or is incapable of understanding biological systems and the true chronic illness process.

PART 4

If God is really transcendent and immanent as He is alleged to be by theologians, it is difficult to logically explain how anything unnatural could be permitted to occur in the universe. Spiritual healers say that God created the universe and all in it from His supreme position superior to all. If such a God directly created man, how could He have created something with unnatural properties? Moreover, if God is immanent and is truly with all creatures all the time, it is again difficult to understand how anything unnatural could occur in the human mind or body.

We are forced to conclude, if we pursue this line of reason, that God is not truly transcendent and immanent; and, therefore, unnatural things occur which He is powerless to stop. If God is not transcendent nor immanent, then the Holy Spirit is not a reliable device to attempt to manipulate for a cure of alleged unnatural problems of mind or body.

If disease is considered to be natural, then we are again forced to conclude that God approves of suffering and disease, is powerless to prevent disease, or is capable of preventing disease but does not care to do so. Thus, it would again seem improvident for the patient to rely upon the Holy Spirit to cure his chronic ailment.

It would appear that the cleric has a vested commercial interest in his role as alleged manipulator of the Holy Spirit, just as any drug doctor, surgeon, or herbal doctor also has his personal vested interest in his own particular line of therapy. It behooves the sufferer to be wary, because many doctors—spiritual, pharmaceutical, or surgical—are apt to overrate their particular brand of therapy and use it in a manner not always in the patient's best interest.

Holy Spirit: If the Holy Spirit is truly supernatural, extra-terrestrial, divinely ethereal, beyond the secular and temporal realm, then it is beyond the ability of man to control. Such an agency is beyond this world and all that is in it.

If the Holy Spirit is controlled by God, then it cannot be controlled by man. For if man could modify the Holy Spirit, man could also modify God. However, man cannot modify God because God is said to be supernatural and transcendent in His omniscience and omnipotence. God is alleged by theists to be one who knows all, and all things which occur do so at His sufferance and pleasure.

It seems that any person who presumes controlling intimacy with such a force is suffering from delusions of grandeur, an arrogance which may be associated with dementia, or false and flagrant assumption of such a role to impress the ignorant and exploit them in a variety of unethical ways.

God's Grace: Figuratively and symbolically speaking, we may safely say that all chronic illness comes from loss of God's Grace. However, this leads to a figurative and symbolic remedy which can have no effect upon real disease of our material body and worldly mind. And, after all, it is the material body and earthly mind that interests Pleneurethic, not a spiritual body which is perfect, hence by definition cannot be manipulated by men. For that which is allegedly inherently perfect in the spiritual and eternal realm is immune to the hand or thought of man, if it were not it would be imperfect.

Theologians misunderstand: Theologians specializing in spiritual healing mistake the source of complete well-being which accompanies the state of perfect health. They attribute it to a special dispensation of God's Grace, when in reality it is ordinary, common, to be enjoyed by anyone who has complete cerebellar sufficiency.

Chronic illness is not due to loss of God's Grace but due instead to loss of bioductory balance and cerebellar sufficiency. Restoration of health is not to be achieved by addressing the Holy Spirit or laying on of sacred hands, but by reestablishing cerebellar sufficiency. Restoration of neural sufficiency must be in operation of this material world since the first cause of the chronic neural disorder sprang from this material world *ab initio*. We speak now only of chronic illness, excluding congenital abnormalities, which are outside the scope of Pleneurethic once they have been formed in the fetus.

Theologians are on untenable ground when they speak of spiritual cure of chronic physical illness. Theologians are free to advocate spiritual cure of spiritual sickness, but when they step over into the temporal world and imply that spiritual sickness causes chronic physical illnesses, acute intellectual distress, or bad behavior, they draw argument from Pleneurethic.

God does not exhibit mal intent: Chronic disease does not result directly from God's mal intent; hence, there is nothing on God's side that needs rectifying by man through supplication in an effort to regain somatic health.

God is alleged to be a supreme person on supernatural level capable of total love; hence, He would not by His own act single out some person and impose suffering by causing the chronic illness process to be established. Since, according to Pleneurethical philosophy, God does not deliberately direct the disease process, He cannot be successfully petitioned to intervene and arrest the course of deteriorating biological affairs at play in chronic illness cases.

God, according to Pleneurethical philosophy, will not personally and directly cause an organ to become painful and break down into purulence. God will not directly cause paralysis, nor will God create a deep and chronic anxiety syndrome to develop without some real direct worldly cause for all of these things. Pleneurethic does not sanction the petition of God to correct some illness He did not cause in the first place. Rather, Pleneurethic addresses itself to worldly causes for chronic illness—all of which can be found in the individual and immediately outside.

In Pleneurethic we do not treat the disease to restore health, but rather we treat the basic cause of the disease. God, the Absolute, does not cause disease; hence, we do not waste time by resorting to fruitless appeals to God to restore health that which He did not cause in the first place.

All healing of chronic physical illness has been said by ministers to be from God. I say, all such healing is from cerebellar sufficiency and other earthly requirements such as nutrition, air, water, etc. If brain capability is destroyed, God is helpless, for He will not even temporarily repeal natural law (established by Him) so as to unnaturally upset the health and sickness process.

After all, what is the loss of one individual compared to the loss of an entire species if the total law would be changed to benefit one particular person in an abnormal situation?

PART 5

The Absolute: The Absolute established laws which permit human form and consciousness to evolve and human individuals to emerge. Human individuals result from an organization of natural forces resident in absolute law mediated by a human neural system and a mentality both of which are also products of absolute law.

The Absolute from its side will not injuriously affect our

neural system or somatic form or mortal mind to cause disease. All human ailments including chronic mental unbalance come from our side—the earthly side—the material world. Treatment of human disease must be addressed to the somatic side, the cerebellar side, the side of the mentality. It cannot be directed at the Absolute's side because there can be no material or worldly trauma from that quarter. The side of the Absolute is perfect, steadfast, undiminished. The only problems that occur are generated by causes on this side—our earthly side—from ignorance, accident, malice of others, bad ethic, etc.

God of Pleneurethic, or the Absolute, if you please, is in His place doing all that He is going to do every split second of every passing minute. We get ill not because of God's abdication of His responsibility, but through our own ignorance, lack of ability to learn, and failure to properly adapt. We get well not because God has changed His mind about letting us be ill, but because we have found the worldly cause for our illness and have corrected the cause.

Prayer and Relaxation: Anything which helps us to psychologically relax will give us a partial assist in reducing the pressure of illness. Although such surface relaxation does not constitute a cure for *chronic tension and illness,* it brings a marked sense of relief to those who hitherto had not learned the secret of relaxation through the use of willpower or resignation.

Prayer, acceptance of God as the ultimate healer, faith in the laying on of hands, etc., all operate to achieve a degree of psychological relaxation through submission or total resignation. Although such antics do not correct the cause of the chronic illness, they do on some occasions help to relieve some acute symptoms disturbing to patient, his associates, and the pseudohealer who wishes to achieve a quick although impermanent victory and win his compensation.

PART 6

Failure of Science: Once a problem is accepted by people as being of spiritual origin, it has been deftly removed from the realm of science and transferred into a precinct definitely under the aegis of spiritual healers. Such a transfer is very easily accomplished when science fails to find the key to chronic illness.

Such is the state of affairs today, for despite the daily press release that a new breakthrough in drug medicine has been accomplished, mature people know that regular healers just cannot cure chronic illness with drugs despite a contrary belief by expertly brainwashed high-school children, perennial college sophomores, etc.

Every mature person knows that drugs do not cure chronic illness; hence, a resurgence of willingness to believe chronic illness to be caused by spiritual affairs. Men who claim competency to cure chronic illness by spiritual manipulation, and actually practice such a theory, know it really does not work— but who cares. Common men are alleged to be thoroughly depraved anyway, and while being fraudulently treated for chronic illness perhaps they can be converted to some organization in need of funds through donations.

State of Mind: Religious healing actually seems based on state of worldly mind; hence, it is more psychotherapeutic than spiritual. With a suitably conditioned religious "state of worldly mind," the sick are alleged to be instantly cured.

State of worldly mind must be the only real basis for religious healing, for that is the only thing that the priest can himself control to any degree. The priest cannot manipulate divine mind. The priest does have competency, through the faith of the ill person, to change the sick person's state of worldly mind, temporarily at best.

"Laying on of sacred hands" as a cure for chronic illness by invoking activity of the Holy Spirit seems illogical. The Holy Spirit is immaterial; hence, the lay on of material hands can in no way be efficacious as far as controlling the Holy Spirit. However, we are faced with evidence that laying on of hands does improve the patient's condition in many instances. Since laying on of hands is not accomplished forcefully or expertly, it cannot reposture bioducts. Its only merit seems this: the laying on of hands, aside from massage value, a symbol of brotherly love and compassion, etc., carries psychological significance if the patient "believes" with fervor and faith. The laying on of hands can have no lasting effect upon the cause of chronic illness, but it can remove some psychological tension, as acute terror and fright are replaced by resignation, belief in an instantaneous cure, or acceptance of one's fate. *In such cases the patient's health has not been restored. He has simply made a good psychological adjustment to his condition by changing his state of mind. How much better it would be if the patient would experience restructuring of his bioductory system and brain so as to permanently restore the basis for health.*

A bad or negative state of mind cannot produce chronic illness by itself, but it can cause real and acute distress whose physical and mental symptoms may be unpleasant. A good or positive state of mind cannot cure chronic illness by itself, because it cannot resurrect the brain or reposture traumatized bioducts, but it can temporarily abate the severity of distressing symptoms of such illness by modifying one's interpretation of such symptoms, and reducing total load on brain capability.

Unjustified and Excessive Optimism: An excessively and unjustifiably negative or positive state of mind is injurious in its violence to an orderly mentality. Most people know of the demerits of an excessively negative state of mind, but they are not so keenly aware of the mischief an inordinately unrealistic positive state of mind can create. An excessively negative state of mind can lead us to suicide or deep despondency because of imagined abuse. An unrealistically positive state of mind can lead to problems stemming from high and unfounded elation over imagined success.

This, then, is my complaint against the false healer, including the spiritual healer. They create an improper positive state of mind and thereby do injury to the patient. They injure the patient because they have not cured the cause of chronic illness. By simply creating an overly optimistic state of mind regarding a false cure, they surreptitiously induce the chronically ill to permit his real ailment to remain untreated.

Thus, the patient is easily exploited, through a form of hypnosis induced by soft-sell advertising, into focusing his faithful attention on such ideas as the notion of instantaneous divine healing of a worldly complaint, ventilation of unclean desire, electrical magnetism, metaphysical prayer, or affirmation of spiritual truth, etc.

Exacerbation, Remission, and the Faith Healer: Most faith healers trade on the principle that chronic illness is usually characterized over the years by a series of exacerbations and remissions of the patient's symptoms. Actually, the real cause of the disease is not fluctuating, it is only the patient's surface symptoms and his interpretation of these symptoms which fluctuate. After each flare-up, the patient seems to recover. This provides the faith healer with fertile ground to work his mysterious and worthless magic.

The faith healer pulls into town, with tinseled tongue and lavish promises, and incites many of the chronically ill with false hope. Charged with a brief flurry of energy from excitement of the moment, plus renewed hope that he can get well, the sufferer rises to the occasion, picks up his bed, and walks. However, the sequel to the story is always the same in real cases of true chronic illness. Within a week or two at most, the spell cast by the itinerant faith healer has subsided, and the sufferer is back to his original desperate condition, having been disillusioned once again. But the tinsel-tongued tout does not know of this or even care, for he is now in the next village, spreading his worthless works.

Thus, the moral of our story is that chronically ill people always seem to recover from every flare-up of their illness except the last one. The faith healer insinuates himself into the series of flare-ups and takes credit for seeming recoveries which could and would have occurred temporarily anyway when the next remission of symptoms was due.

Major Problem: The major problem in regular healing today is that for nearly all the cases of chronic illness, the regular drug physician does not know where to find the structural cause of chronic illness within the patient. Since they are ignorant of the cause of chronic mental and physical illness they say none exists.

The stage is thereby set for a field day among the preachers of the Gospel who happen to decide they want to practice their own strange and particular brand of nebulous faith healing on chronic illness. We cannot call them all charlatans by intent, but they certainly are opportunists who, being improperly prepared, cause much additional suffering than need be.

APPENDIX 3
Guilt

PART 1

Restoration of health, by application of Pleneurethical measures, often requires that the symptom of intense guilt be understood.

To understand the Pleneurethical method of analyzing the problem of guilt, we must divide it into at least two classes; simple or acute guilt, and complex or chronic guilt.

First key to guilt: we ourselves must feel we have done something wrong. Or we must take responsibility for that which is imagined wrong, and for which we believe ourselves to be somehow related.

Guilt is a personal thing. Even if we have done no wrong, but believe we have, we will feel guilty. Or perhaps we have committed a perfectly repugnant crime, but we feel no guilt, unless we later feel it to have been wrong.

Preachers and parole officers may berate the wrongdoer regularly, telling him he should feel guilty and repent. But all such prattle may have little effect upon the intransigent, who more than likely feels he has been exceedingly clever.

PART 2

Simple guilt is psychological and comes at us through our belief alone. We believe we must go to Sunday school to be virtuous, but we go fishing instead and here is the basis for simple guilt. Or we believe the duty of man is to protect woman, but we drown a woman as we drive her off the side of a pier in our powerful black sedan. Here again is the basis for simple guilt.

The thing about simple guilt is that on the day we decide to analyze its real meaning and shrug it off our shoulders, or rather off our brain, we will immediately be free of its depressing weight. It may take a little longer on some occasions than others to rationalize away our simple guilt but it can be and usually is done.

In simple or acute guilt the central neurological system remains chronically unimpaired. It may be acutely overloaded from time to time, but its basic neurological tissue capability has not deteriorated, pathologically and chronically. Hence, the basic ingredient for sustained mental and physical health prevails. Once the disagreeable social, economic, or academic episode has passed and a psychological adjustment made, complete recovery from the feeling of guilt is possible. This is especially true if ventilative and other techniques are employed to remove all lingering traces that may have been repressed in the deepest reach of the conscious mind.

There are many experts around to help us in our task. Preachers, psychiatrists, psychologists, hypnotists, and all others like them are willing to aid in such a venture.

Another very significant aspect of simple and acute guilt is that the emotion felt by the person is not uniformly related to any specific wrongful act. A gangster may accept a contract to murder another person. Upon completion of the contract he may feel no depressive guilt but elation instead as he collects his wages and heads for the bank. However, the same gangster may feel guilt if he holds out on his wife and family. Or a senator that drowns his girl friend may feel little guilt, but concern instead for his career and how to shift the onus for his act to the shoulders of another.

PART 3

And now we come to complex or chronic guilt. This form of guilt was never before recognized until my Pleneurethical writing revealed it, outlined its connection with other classes of guilt, and related it to the chronic anxiety syndrome.

Prior to Pleneurethic, the form of guilt I now discuss was uncritically considered to be just another form of simple guilt—hence, amenable to a rational or mystical approach on a verbal, metaphysical, or idealistic level of communication.

First key to chronic guilt! the sufferer actually has been involved, whether he remembers it or not, in something anatomically wrong and heavily traumatic. There is real trouble within his body. But the trouble springs not from a traumatic psychological event in mind which can be analyzed in terms of structure of intellect nor even from such an acute disturbance as a broken arm. Rather, it comes from trouble of a traumatic physiological nature which causes chronic bioductory malstructure, and is altogether a chronic cerebellar tissue disturbance and not a psychological misadventure.

Chronic guilt is pervasive and persistent. The brain tissue is chronically depleneurized from submental attack and conflict. The cerebellar vitality required for sustained mental and physical health has been forfeited to some physical traumatic accident to the bioductory system in the past. A heavy fall from the crib, a drunken obstetrician complete with arrogant attitude and obstreperous steel clamps, or an athletic field necksnap or fall from a horse are enough to call it into being. Harsh words in themselves will never call it into being, nor will any psychological misadventure.

Chronic guilt, then, is aroused by chronic physical trauma to the bioductory system which mechanically harasses and depresses central neurological tissues, especially the brain. The fact that chronic guilt is basically a physioneurological mechanism, and not exclusively a psychological mechanism, is of great significance, in my Pleneurethical view. Had I not made this breakthrough in thought some years ago, Pleneurethic would never have been created.

In chronic guilt, the sufferer knows that something is wrong within. There is a vague internal uneasiness as if the person had committed a wrongful act which the person acknowledges to have been wrong, hence has the ingredient for the emotion of guilt. In chronic guilt there is often a heavy self-reproach manifested to match the severity of the neurological turbulence and tension generated by the chronic depleneurizing tensions.

Punishment is another companion of guilt. Early in life we learn that if we are guilty of infringing the family law, punishment is the result. Most persons then associate guilt and punishment in the same mental picture. Inner duress, created by the chronic depleneurizing process of brain tissue from severe neuralosis, may be interpreted by the sufferer as punishment. The feeling of punishment may be very strong, although the source of the penalty may not be apparent to the sufferer.

And while I speak of the punishment meted out to a suffering person by his neuralosis and its depleneurizing effect on brain tissues—let me say, it is real suffering. It is not imagined by the sufferer, despite what the professors and physicians say. It is real, and it is the hidden reason for so much academic consternation and so many perplexed scientists, when they try to correlate results of various biological tests on human guinea pigs. Very often, in a random sampling of people chosen for biological tests, there will be a substantial number of people with moderate or even severe chronic depleneurization of cerebellar tissues. The presence of these people injects a skew into the laboratory test that is not taken into consideration by the scientists in the laboratory.

Personal adjustment to acute and chronic guilt is vastly different on the self-help level. Now in simple guilt, the necessary psychological adjustment is made relatively easily. We admonish ourselves not to do it again or throw a good drunk, and we are free from our mental fetters.

But when chronic guilt unrelentingly grips us, and we feel the callous force of it for a lifetime—even though we attempt repeatedly to escape—we feel ourselves caught in some evil and mysterious circumstance. Such a person readily believes, if told by others, that an evil spell has been cast upon him by the Devil or Holy Spirit. He is open to suggestion that the evil spell may be dismissed only through counterspiritual offensive by the village medicine man, community minister, or neighborhood psychiatric healer.

Chronic guilt, being physiological and of central neurological genesis, is part of the other half of the degenerative disease syndrome. In the beginning of the chronic central neurological irregularity, which eventually leads to severe brain depression and the emotion of abject guilt, there may be brain irritation that causes the emotion of extreme excitement and exhilaration. The mechanism of chronic guilt is often masked in initial stages by a vivacious temperament.

Guilt may be classified and analyzed clearly in the classroom according to source, but in the individual experiencing the guilt it is seldom clear cut. The small boy who disobeys his mother's command not to leave the house but does so anyway, because he cannot resist the call of the apples in the nearby orchard, suffers guilt because he feels he has violated his mother's trust. And the guilt is reinforced by the acute neural distress from green apple indigestion. However, such guilt vanishes automatically after the green apples have passed through his intestinal tract and the guilty emotion from disobedience of mother's orders has been psychologically ventilated through some childish rationalization.

Or, as another example, a once very proper and responsible person loses his competence because of a football field accident which has now depleneurized his brain and ruined his character. He no longer acts properly, he flares up in intense anger over small incidents, and even exhibits generally poor judgment from the spur of his uncontrolled emotions. Upon reviewing the incidents of the day, the person feels guilty because of his improper behavior. So here we have an underlying chronic guilt feeling from a depleneurized central neural system, reinforced psychologically by imprudent outbursts of temper or exhibitions of general incompetence which he later realizes to have been wrong.

Constant emotion of guilt for which the afflicted can assign no specific rational cause, or a cause that shifts from day to day, is a symptom of possible chronic brain trauma of bioductory origin. The person who feels guilt because he neglected to insure the home—and his family now suffers—has a rational and simple cause to feel guilt. But the Arab immigrant to the United States who, after falling on his head from a horse, feels guilt because he has not yet killed a senator thought to be causing all the trouble for the Arabs, is reflecting a chronic mental illness and emotion of guilt for which there is no psychological cure. He may be counseled out of his feeling of guilt, and chronic hostility toward a certain senator, but he will simply project it in another direction later on—unless the chronic source of his brain depleneurization is corrected by Pleneurethical biomechanical operation.

APPENDIX 4

The basic mechanism of Pleneurethical thought is desire to accept responsibility for proper execution of one's own ethical affairs, intellectual development, and physical well-being. This is the law of Pleneurethic, all else being but rhetorical expansion.

Shifting the blame for failure of self, to someone or something external to the individual, is a basic malmechanism of thought. Even an entire generation may engage in a mass shifting of responsibility for alleged failure to achieve the good life, for example, the modern generation damning the preceding generation for all its ills, real and imagined.

The Pleneurethical mind is not malicious, nor does it endeavor to belittle or overcome the mind of another person. It will strive vigorously and resolutely to test theories. It will impeach irrelevancy of principle, and joust with kniving institutions; but there is one thing it will never do in premeditation. The Pleneurethical mind will never trifle with another person.

Preservation of the dignity of every person and animal is a fundamental tenet of Pleneurethic. No one ever violates another person's dignity or comfort in any witting way and remains a serious student of Pleneurethic. Rape is out, so is taking another's property without his permission, as is loud talk, loud music in quiet neighborhoods, and all other such nuisances. Depression of mental buoyance in another person by some cutting phrase is also to be avoided. We should refuse to even develop the capability for such verbal combat.

To be Pleneurethical, we must observe the fundamental worth of every other living being, young or old, firm or infirm. Each person has a right to conscientious search for a proper role in life.

True dignity, springing from inner ethical consciousness and wisdom, is what the serious student cultivates in Pleneurethic.

Pleneurethic would solve the world's problems by teaching character development first, and by instruction in art and science and trade second. For what real and lasting benefit to the world is a highly tutored but unprincipled individual, who uses his license and expertise as a device to cheat and deceive the people? The lowering of the level of public health is inestimable because of the unprincipled opportunists who defraud the people.

GLOSSARY

ABSOLUTE   Prime source of all force that prevails behind the grid of absolute law from which our universe is elaborated.

ABSOLUTE LAW   Basic array of force from which our universe is draped. From the network of force, which stands as a buffer between our universe and the first source, or absolute principle, such things are derived as mass, temperature, velocity, space, orbit, light, consciousness, life.

ANXIETY   Worry, apprehension and mental torment with accompanying somatic symptoms.

ANXIETY, acute   Derives chiefly from acute disorder in the brain caused by psychological disorder and malstructuring of the intellect from fear of a psychological derivation.

ANXIETY, chronic   Derives from chronic disorder in the brain caused by chronic injury to the bioductory system tissues in the more cephalward portions of the system.

ARAM   A principle of absolute law—the animatory force of nature.

ARAMIFICATION   Animation of material by Aramic force to produce an individual of any species now or to evolve later.

BIODUCTORY SYSTEM   Protective environment of ducts which encloses the brain and the remainder of the neural system.

BIODUCTOSIS   Chronic disorder in the bioductory system and immediate adjacent area. First cause of chronic illness process.

BRAIN   The central structure of man. Brain absorbs tension and reflects this stress to its several coaxial structures.

BRAIN SYSTEM   Brain, spinal cord, and peripheral neural system. It is anatomically coextensive and coaxial with the bioductory system.

COAXIALITY   The structure of the brain is related to the structure of mind, body and the outside world.

DEPLENEURIZE   Debilitating process that reduces brain competence.

DREAM   A neuromental process during sleep associated with reduction of brain tension caused by mental efforts involved in events of preceding day or days.

DREAM, day   Undisciplined neuromental process while awake to reduce ordinary cerebellar tension.

FUNCTION   Activity generated by an operating structure.

HEALTH   A spontaneous biological process promoted and fostered by unimpaired brain structure and function.

ILLNESS, acute   Caused by vectors other than those responsible for chronic brain disturbance. Generally heals with passage of time.

ILLNESS, chronic   Condition caused by degenerative disturbance or injury to the brain from bioductosis. Will not cure itself.

ILLNESS, congenital   Derives from permanent brain defect occurring during gestation.

INFRALLECT or infraconsciousness   Associated with that part of the brain's activity which presides over the operation of the visceral and vascular body segments.

INFRALLECTOSIS   Malstructure of the infrallect through hypnosis, habitual denial, or discouragement of specific body functions.

INTELLECT or intellectual consciousness   That sector of the mentality devoted to ordinary conscious activity and thought.

INTELLECTOSIS   Malstructure of the belief structure of the intellect. Intellectosis with its mental conflict may acutely depleneurize cerebellar tissues.

MENTALITY   Product of interaction between brain and mind. Interpretation by mind of brain performance.

MENTOSIS   Reflection of neuralosis on the mind to produce chronic mental illness and chronic anxiety.

NEURALOSIS   Chronic stress in central neural system, especially the brain, caused by bioductosis which causes chronic illness.

NIGHTMARE   Interpretation by the mind of turbulent cerebellar activity during sleep produced by chronic neurological trauma and tension resulting from physical injury to the bioductory system.

PLENEURETHIC   Study of mankind and his environment from the standpoint of the structure of the individual's brain and peripheral neural system—its capabilities, limitations, and requirements.

PLENEURIZE   Bringing the brain to optimum competence.

PROCESS, chronic illness   Continuing deterioration of mental and physical resources due to chronic brain problems. There will be characteristic exacerbations and remissions plus shifting of symptom patterns throughout the history and maturation of the ailment.

REPLENEURIZE   Restoration of brain integrity and capability by reversing the course of the contributing neuralosis.

SOMA   The body, especially the parts separate from the brain and its neural system.

SOMATOSIS   Chronic illness in body tissues from neuralosis, variable according to the pattern of stresses.

STRESS   Stress accumulates in the brain, leading to its structural distortion (either micro, macro, or both) and causes mental and physical disease concurrently.

STRUCTURE   Structural configuration controls functional characteristics. Stressful distortion of structure adversely affects functional capability. Disease results.

SURI'S TRACT   Nerve cell section in the brain and associated tracts influencing the operation of the vascular system servicing the brain.

TIME   A biological phenomenon resulting from conscious interaction between a mind and a functioning brain. In coma or periods of unconsciousness, the sense of the passage of time is repealed because mind is not conscious of brain activity or transpiration of external events.

ULTRALLECT or ultraconsciousness   That portion of the mind above the level of ordinary day-to-day thinking. The immediate inspirational source of our ethical and moral nature.

ULTRALLECTOSIS   Distortion of the structure of normal ethical awareness by coaching of others who are morally unfit, unethical autosuggestions.